J. Théron   J. Moret

Spinal Phlebography

Lumbar and Cervical Techniques

With the Collaboration of

D. Dilenge, J.P. Houtteville

and   H. Ammerich   P. Blanchot   D. Chevalier   A. Chevrot
J. F. Ginestie   D. Larde   L. Picard   J. Roland   J. Vignaud

With a Foreword by R. Djindjian

With 113 Figures in 182 Separate Illustrations

Springer-Verlag Berlin Heidelberg New York 1978

The cover picture is a schematic drawing of the *lumbar epidural veins on an AP phlebogram* which is shown in more detail in Figure 16 on page 30.

ISBN 3-540-08867-9 Springer-Verlag Berlin Heidelberg New York
ISBN 0-387-08867-9 Springer-Verlag New York Heidelberg Berlin

Library of Congress Cataloging in Publication Data. Théron, Jacques, 1943–. Spinal phlebography (lumbar and cervical techniques). Bibliography: p. Includes index. 1. Spinal cord – Blood-vessels – Radiography. 2. Spine – Blood-vessels – Radiography. 3. Veins – Radiography. I. Moret, Jaques, 1947– joint author. II. Dilenge, Domenico. III. Title. RC400.T43 616.8′7 78-18285

Reproduction of the figures: Gustav Dreher GmbH, Stuttgart

Monophoto typesetting, printing, and bookbinding: Universitätsdruckerei H. Stürtz AG, Würzburg
2123/3130–543210

Foreword and Historical Review

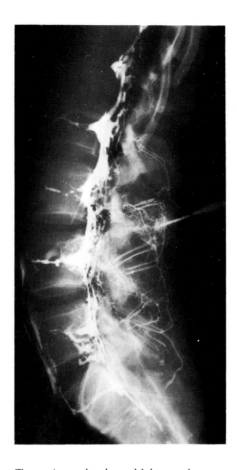

Transpinous lumbar phlebography performed on a specimen. Lateral projection. (Professor R. DJINDJIAN, 1958)

In the 1950s, understanding of vertebromedullary pathology could only benefit from a new means of information and it was logical to investigate new techniques, the results of which could be compared to the neuroradiologic techniques used at that time: Lipiodol or air myelography and Methiodal radiculography. Phlebography was the first vascular neuroradiologic technique for the spine. Inspired by pelvic phlebography, performed by transpubic injection [33], and by phlebography of the legs by transcalcanean injection [56], FISCHGOLD et al. in 1952 [40] injected Diodone into the lumbar spinous processes. They found opacification of the epidural veins, and compared the films to the anatomic drawings by BRESCHET (1829) [11]. In 1956, ROUSSEAU and GOURNET [74] studied in specimens, in dogs, and finally in man the normal opacification of the epidural venous system. They named this technique "transspinous phlebography of the spine." In 1958, we personally began using phlebography and later tried to replace the puncture of the spinous process by cavography; we tested the technique in various spinal conditions using simultaneous AP and lateral seriography and the subtraction technique. This work was continued from 1959 to 1961 [28, 29, 31] with the collaboration of P. BAGET [7] and P. DORLAND and A. PANSINI.

At this time our conclusions were that phlebography was a "perfect" technique for demonstrating the venous vascularization of the spine. Its results in the diagnosis of tumoral or traumatic lesions and in disc herniations were compared to those of methiodal radiculography and checked surgically; we found phlebography to be a technique of great promise, but its practicability needed to be determined by more extensive experimental research.

Naturally, this technique was also applied to the investigation of the spinal angiomas, because it seemed logical when confronted with vascular anomalies to try to obtain their opacification. In fact all attempts failed and we demonstrated only dilated venous spinal plexuses that corresponded to the pictures observed on the late phase of the subsequently developed spinal cord arteriograms. In March 1961, J. LEFEBVRE and C. FAURE asked us to perform spinal phlebography on a young patient who had had several subarachnoid hemorrhages; carotid and vertebral angiograms were normal. Spinal phlebography showed only minor anomalies. We were not aware of any direct opacification of a spinal cord angioma, but our knowledge of arteriovenous fistulas encouraged us to attempt opacification of the malformation via the arterial approach. Aortography using a femoral approach was performed at the same time as the phlebography and showed for the first time an angioma of the thoracolumbar spinal cord. Spinal cord arteriography was born and we went on to develop its possibilities for the study of angiomas, tumors, and ischemic disorders. Conversely, this caused us to abandon spinal phlebography.

Nevertheless this technique was further developed in Italy [60], in the United States [77], in England [50], and in West Germany [90]. Techniques of puncture of spinous processes were developed along with phlebography by catheterization of the iliac veins with abdominal compression [48] and of the ascending lumbar vein [12–14, 41, 57, 64, 72, 89]. JACQUES THÉRON, in the department of Neuroradiology of the Lariboisière Hospital, has developed catheterization of the ascending lumbar veins and also of the lateral sacral veins, which permits better opacification of the epidural venous system; in 1976 in collaboration with Dr. JACQUES MORET of the Rothschild Foundation, he designed a very accurate and very reliable technique, which is now in daily use. In 1973 he also developed a technique of opacification of the cervical epidural veins by catheterization of the vertebral veins, which has now replaced the classic technique by puncture of a vertebral body described by GREITZ in 1962.

Spinal phlebography thus represents a great step forward in the neuroradiologic diagnosis of disc herniations but also in many other spinal conditions in which myelography and angiography had limitations. It is not too much to say that Professeur Agrégé J. THÉRON, Doctor J. MORET, and their collaborators have been completely successful in the publication of this monograph, which is of great credit to the French School of Neuroradiology. I am personally particularly happy to present this work, which reflects their tenacity and their dedication to neuroradiology.

Hôpital Lariboisière
Paris, July 1st 1977   Professor RENÉ DJINDJIAN

Preface

Spinal phlebography is an "indirect" radiologic technique for investigating vertebromedullary pathology. It is a harmless and almost painless technique that does not require the introduction of contrast medium into the subarachnoid spaces. Its interpretation is based on the modifications of the epidural veins which do not themselves have any proven pathology.

The longitudinal epidural veins are situated in the anterolateral angles of the spinal canal between the nerve root and the intervertebral disc. They consequently represent a major anatomic landmark in the investigation of disc pathology because they are compressed by a disc herniation before the corresponding nerve root is reached.

The improvement of the techniques of lumbar phlebography by catheterization of the lateral sacral veins and of cervical phlebography by catheterization of the vertebral veins now permits opacification of the epidural venous system along the total length of the lumbar and cervical spine. Spinal phlebography can consequently be used routinely, primarily in disc pathology but now also in other fields of vertebromedullary pathology such as myelopathy, tumors, or stenosis of the spinal canal, where it provides new information as compared to the other techniques of investigation.

The technique and results of spinal phlebography in these various conditions are presented in this monograph which is an attempt, with the collaboration of several authors, to summarize current knowledge in this field.

Only lumbar and cervical phlebography will be discussed in this monograph. Thoracic phlebography is not of the same major interest because of the generally high degree of reliability of the techniques of investigation in this area.

Finally, the reader is sure to be moved when he reads the Foreword and Historival Review by Professor DJINDJIAN, who died only a few weeks after writing it. He was a pioneer of spinal phlebography, and the improvement in the accuracy of the anatomic data obtained, if necessary, by a multiplicity of techniques of investigation, provided that they were efficient and harmless, was always his goal. The authors of this monograph share the same opinion and believe that good treatment can be obtained only by a precise preliminary determination of the location, extent, and nature of a pathologic lesion.

J. THÉRON and J. MORET

Acknowledgments

We wish to thank Prof. A. WACKENHEIM, without whom the publication of this monograph would not have been possible. We also wish to thank the physicians who put their trust in us, even in the early days of our experience, by referring patients for phlebography, in particular Prof. Ag. H. ADAM, Prof. Ag. J.H. AUBRIOT, Dr. N. CARUEL, Dr. Y. CHAOUAT, Prof. Ag. J. COPHIGNON, Prof. R. HOUDART, Prof. Ag. J.P. HOUTTEVILLE, Prof. Ag. B. LECHEVALIER, Dr. J.L. L'HIRONDEL, Prof. Ag. G. LOYAU, Dr. F. MIKOL, Prof. P. MORIN, Prof. Ag. A. REY, Dr. M. SACHS, Dr. Cl. THUREL, Dr. J. VABRET, Dr. C. VIELPEAU. Without their help lumbar and cervical phlebography would not have become the routine techniques that they are today. We are grateful to Mr. C. LALLENEC and Mr. P. ACKER for their photographic work, Mrs. C. BOURDAUD'HUI, Mrs. C. CRUCHON, and Mrs. S. NICOLLE for their help and secretarial assistance in the preparation of the monograph, and the teams of technicians for their daily help with the phlebographies.

J. THÉRON and J. MORET

Contents

Authors and Collaborators

THÉRON, J., Professeur Agrégé, Chef du Service de Neuroradiologie et Radiologie Générale, C.H.U. Clémenceau, F-14000 Caen

MORET, J., Chef de Service-Adjoint, Service de Radiologie, Fondation Ophtalmologique Adolphe de Rothschild, F-75019 Paris

AMMERICH, H., Assistant, Service de Neuroradiologie et Radiologie Pédiatrique, C.H.U. de Strasbourg, F-67005 Strasbourg

BLANCHOT, P., Attaché, Service de Neuroradiologie, C.H.U. de Nancy, F-54000 Nancy

CHEVALIER, D., Interne, Service de Neuroradiologie et Radiologie Générale, C.H.U. Clémenceau, F-14000 Caen

CHEVROT, A., Chef de Clinique-Assistant, Service de Radiologie, C.H.U. Cochin, F-75019 Paris

DILENGE, D., Professeur Titulaire et Directeur du Département de Radiologie Diagnostique, C.H.U. de Sherbrooke, Sherbrooke, Quebec, Canada

GINESTIE, J.F., Radiologiste, Ex-Chef de Clinique, Clinique St. Jean, Avenue Buisson Bertrand, F-34000 Montpellier

HOUTTEVILLE, J.P., Professeur Agrégé, Service de Neurochirurgie, C.H.U. Clémenceau, F-14000 Caen

LARDE, D., Interne, Service de Neuroradiologie, C.H.U. de Nancy, F-54000 Nancy

PICARD, L., Professeur Agrégé, Chef du Service de Neuroradiologie, C.H.U. de Nancy, F-54000 Nancy

ROLAND, J., Médecin Adjoint, Service de Neuroradiologie, C.H.U. de Nancy, F-54000 Nancy

Chapter 1

The Physiologic Role of the Meningorachidian Plexus

D. Dilenge

In the venous circulation, the vertebral venous plexus, which is both intra- and paravertebral, occupies a distinctive place. As it is almost valveless and communicates directly with both vena cavas, superior and inferior, it is one of the most important anastomotic network in the body [8]. This vertebral venous plexus is known by a variety of names, including "meningorachidian plexus" (MRP).

1.1. Anastomotic Availability

The efficiency of this anastomotic network is easily shown at the level of the inferior vena cava, where an obstruction (thrombosis, tumor compression or infiltration, etc.) leads to a shunting of the distal venous blood to the vertebral plexus and, hence, through the azygos vein to the superior vena cava. Figure 1 is an example of this phenomenon, resulting from a hypernephroma. The injection of contrast medium into the distal inferior vena cava clearly outlines the vertebral plexus, particularly in its intravertebral part.

Manual compression of the inferior vena cava below the renal veins produces the same results (Fig. 2) and is one of the ways presently available to demonstrate angiographically the lumbar part of the vertebral plexus. The effect of such compression is dramatic in the monkey, where the injection of 3 cc contrast medium is enough to demonstrate the vertebral plexus as far as the neck, the azygos vein, and the right side of the heart (Fig. 3).

Furthermore, a simple Valsalva maneuver is enough to develop the same shunting. Indeed, it is possible to demonstrate angiographically the diversion of the blood flow from the inferior vena cava to the vertebral venous plexus in man during the Valsalva maneuver. The increased abdominal pressure seems to block the contrast medium in the inferior vena cava at level of the diaphragm (Fig. 4).

1.2. Relationships with the Jugular System

In spite of the well-known existence of extensive anastomoses linking this plexus to the sinuses of the base of the skull and to the jugular veins, its functional role in the cerebral circulation is little known.

We have confirmed the important relationship of this plexus to the cerebral circulation in our first series of 25 experiments, in twelve Macacus rhesus monkeys. We observed that in jugular vein obstruction, the entire cerebral venous return reaches the superior vena cava via the vertebral plexus. After compressing the jugular veins with a tourniquet, the injection of contrast medium into an internal jugular vein, above the compression, clearly demonstrates the cervical part of the vertebral plexus (Fig. 5). Applying this technique in man [27], we were able to demonstrate this plexus in the cervical region (Fig. 6).

These experiments not only confirm the presence of rich anastomoses between the vertebral plexus and surrounding venous structures in the area of the foramen magnum but they also suggest the existence of an important function of the vertebral plexus in the cerebral circulation.

1.3. The Meningorachidian Plexus (MRP) as a Main Pathway of Cerebral Venous Return

With regard to this physiologic role we have noted, during routine cerebral angiography in man, some hemodynamic characteristics of cerebral venous drainage. In the majority of instances the opafication of the intracranial sinuses was followed by filling either one or both internal jugular veins. In certain instances the opacification of the intracranial sinuses was also followed by the opacification of the vertebral plexus; in these cases, opacification of the internal jugular vein was partial (Fig. 7a) or absent (Fig. 7b). In still fewer instances, where the filling of the vertebral plexus seemed extensive, the opacification of the internal jugular vein was barely noticeable (Fig. 7c).

1.4. The Postural Phenomenon [25]

We later studied both experimentally and clinically the role of the vertebral plexus in cerebral venous return during changes in the position of the body (Fig. 5). With the animal supine, contrast medium injected into a jugular vein goes mostly, or entirely, into the internal and external jugular veins (Fig. 5a). When the injection is repeated with the animal upright, the medium goes mostly or almost exclusively to the vertebral plexus (Fig. 5c). Sometimes, the jugular veins and the plexus are demonstrated simultaneously; but with the animal supine, the jugular system is always better demonstrated; conversely, in the upright position, it is the vertebral plexus that is best filled.

The same phenomenon was observed in man (Fig. 8). The internal jugular vein is well shown following the injection of 10 cc contrast medium in the upper part of the jugular vein in the decubitus position. When the injection is repeated with the patient in the sitting position, the internal jugular vein is less well outlined, but the vertebral plexus with the paravertebral and epidural veins are demonstrated [27].

In order to observe this phenomenon under optimal physiologic conditions, we injected the contrast medium into the aortic arch of the monkey and followed the circulation of the dye through the venous phase. In the supine animal, the medium appears in the jugular veins only (Fig. 9a). With the animal upright, the vertebral plexus is demonstrated (Fig. 9b). We have confirmed the existence of this postural phenomenon in man under similar conditions, during both carotid and vertebral arteriography (Fig. 10). These observations provide conclusive evidence that the vertebral venous plexus can be an important and sometimes exclusive pathway for cerebral venous return.

EPSTEIN and co-workers [37] have also described this postural phenomenon by injecting contrast medium into the intracranial venous sinuses of monkeys.

1.5. The Postural Phenomenon at the Level of the Inferior Vena Cava [25]

The explanation for the effect of body position on the pathway of cerebral venous return remains a largely unanswered question. We are currently attempting to solve this problem but it would appear that the explanation is not related to anatomic or physiologic conditions that are specific to the craniocervical region. Indeed, we have found that a similar postural phenomenon exists at the level of the inferior vena cava. This is seen following injection of the common iliac vein, which opacified almost exclusively the vertebral plexus in the absence of compression of the vena cava, when the animal is hanging vertically with the head down (Fig. 11). In man, THERON [81] also showed very distinct opacification of the vertebral venous plexus during the injection of the contrast medium into the iliac vein, without abdominal compression, with the patient in the vertical position, head down (Fig. 12).

It may be that the passage of blood through various levels of the MRP is largely determined by changes in the caliber of the spinal dural sac which occur with changes in body position.

Alternatively, the lack of flow in the internal jugular vein in the upright position may be due to its collapse when its intraluminal pressure becomes negative.

1.6. Increased Intrathoracic Pressure

In another series of experiments, we studied the relationship that may exist between intrathoracic pressure and cerebral venous flow [42]. Since the cerebral venous return passes through the chest cavity, it may be affected by changes in thoracic pressure. The effect of body position on cerebral blood flow was also studied in relation to changes in intrathoracic pressure in an attempt to determine the respective importance of the vertebral plexus and the jugular system under such conditions.

The first experimental step consisted in an angiographic study in the monkey. Contrast medium was injected into the internal jugular vein in various body positions with normal breathing and under conditions of increased intrathoracic pressure (60–130 cm of water). The angiographic findings are illustrated in Figure 13.

When the animals are subjected to high intrathoracic pressure, in the decubitus position (A) the jugular veins are seen to be distended at the end of inspiration. The contrast medium appears to be blocked at the entrance into the chest. The vertebral plexus is seen but is not injected below C7. In the upright position however (B) the jugular veins are less well shown and the vertebral plexus becomes the major pathway of drainage; in fact, it is better filled and is visible down to below the level of the heart. Jugular venous return obstruction appears to be compensated through the cervical vertebral venous plexus, this compensation being more efficient in the upright position.

Following these morphologic observations, we attempted to confirm the existence, and to document the extent, of the compensatory mechanism offered by the vertebral plexus. This was done by measuring the cerebral blood flow in eight monkeys after intracarotid injection of Xenon 133 with the external carotid artery ligated. Arterial blood gases, blood pressure, endotracheal pressure, and intracranial pressure were monitored throughout.

Diagram 1 shows the relation between cerebral blood flow and the $PaCO_2$. The 64 measurements of cerebral blood flow are divided into four experimental groups according to the intrathroacic pressure and the body position. There is a linear regression in the first three groups (normal ventilation in decubitus, normal ventilation standing, and high intrathoracic pressure in decubitus). The regression is not so pronounced in the last group with high thoracic pressure in the standing position.

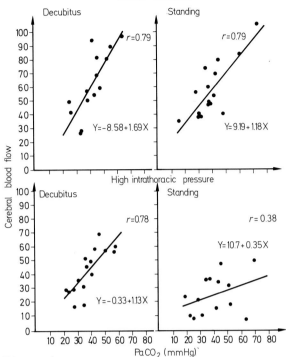

Diagram 1

The slopes of the first and second group are not statistically significant, indicating that the response of the cerebral circulation to CO_2 is not influenced by normal ventilation or body position. When intrathoracic pressure is increased, however, there is a significant difference between the slopes in the standing and the decubitus positions. It would seem, therefore, that the cerebral vessels do not respond normally to CO_2 when there is increased intrathoracic pressure in the standing position.

We then studied the autoregulation of the cerebral circulation under conditions of increased thoracic pressure. This autoregulation is the response of the cerebral blood flow to changes in cerebral perfusion pressure. As seen in Diagram 2, autoregulation is lost earlier in the standing than in the decubitus position when cerebral perfusion pressure de-

5

creases. Furthermore, the two slopes are different once autoregulation is lost.

Analysis of these results indicates that under conditions of increased intrathoracic pressure, the upright position interferes with the compensatory mechanisms of the cerebral circulation in spite of the possible compensation offered by the vertebral plexus.

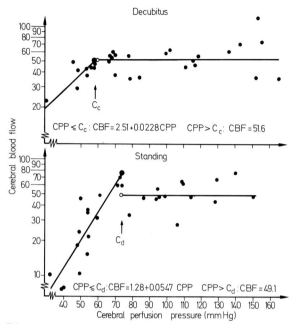

Decubitus

$CPP \leq C_c$: $CBF = 2.51 + 0.0228\,CPP$ $CPP > C_c$: $CBF = 51.6$

Standing

$CPP \leq C_d$: $CBF = 1.28 + 0.0547\,CPP$ $CPP > C_d$: $CBF = 49.1$

Cerebral blood flow

Cerebral perfusion pressure (mmHg)

Diagram 2

Obviously, one must be cautious in interpreting these results. First, our experiments involve a relatively small number of animals; secondly, other important factors such as cardiac output and cerebral metabolism were not measured. However, if these results are reliable, one wonders if one function of the vertebral plexus is not to reduce the untoward effects of increased intrathoracic pressure in the upright position. Indeed, as we have seen, under such conditions, the jugular pathway is obstructed while the vertebral pathway is functional on the angiograms.

1.7. Conclusions

1. Anastomotic shunting via the MRP appears to be the most significant of the entire venous system, permitting free passage of blood from the territory of one vena cava to that of the other. This shunting also takes place under physiologic conditions such as during the Valsalva maneuver.

2. The MRP is a major pathway of cerebral venous return which appears to be just as important as the jugular veins. Indeed, while late films in routine cerebral angiography usually demonstrate the jugular veins, the vertebral plexus is also sometimes seen, either in conjunction with the jugular veins or even, more rarely, instead of the jugular veins.

3. The anastomotic plexus, which is particularly well developed in the area of the foramen magnum, provides a ready compensating mechanism for the least degree of obstruction in the jugular veins. This is easily demonstrated in the course of jugular venography when external compression is applied to the veins below the site of injection.

4. Change in body position is one determining factor that may direct blood flow through the jugular or vertebral systems as alternate routes of cerebral venous return. Studies of this postural phenomenon in the monkey and in man by arteriography and venography have shown that the vertebral plexus tends to become the preferred route of cerebral venous return when the body assumes the upright position.

5. This effect of posture on the course of venous return is not exclusive to the craniocervical region, since venous blood is also shunted from the inferior vena cava to the vertebral plexus when the body is placed vertically with the head down.

6. When intrathoracic pressure is markedly increased, the upright position appears to interfere with the normal response of the cerebral circulation to CO_2. It also seems to interfere with the autoregulation of cerebral circulation, but this untoward effect is possibly somewhat diminished by the presence of the vertebral plexus, which becomes the major pathway of cerebral venous return and may compensate for jugular venous obstruction.

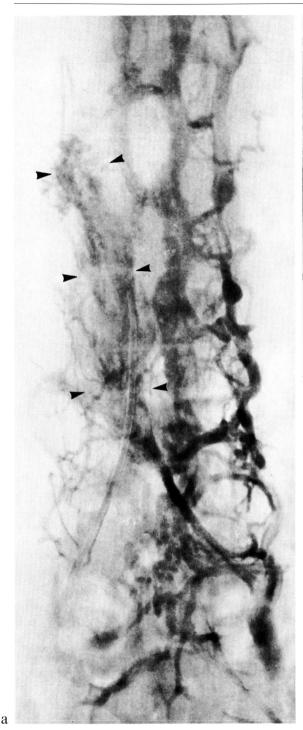

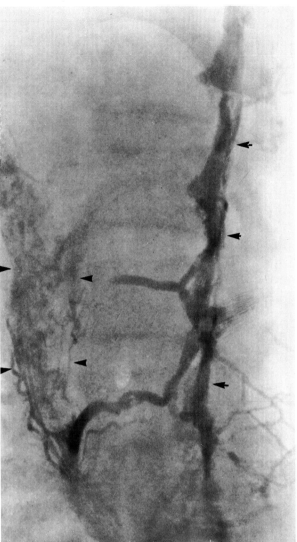

b

Figure 1a (AP view) and b (lateral view)

Venography of inferior vena cava by transfemoral catheter. The vena cava *(arrowheads)* is irregular and poorly
seen because of infiltration and compression by a right-
sided hypernephroma. Contrast medium passes easily into
the lumbar meningorachidian plexus which it clearly outlines, particularly in its intravertebral portion [*arrows* in
(b)] before reaching the azygos vein and the superior vena
cava

a

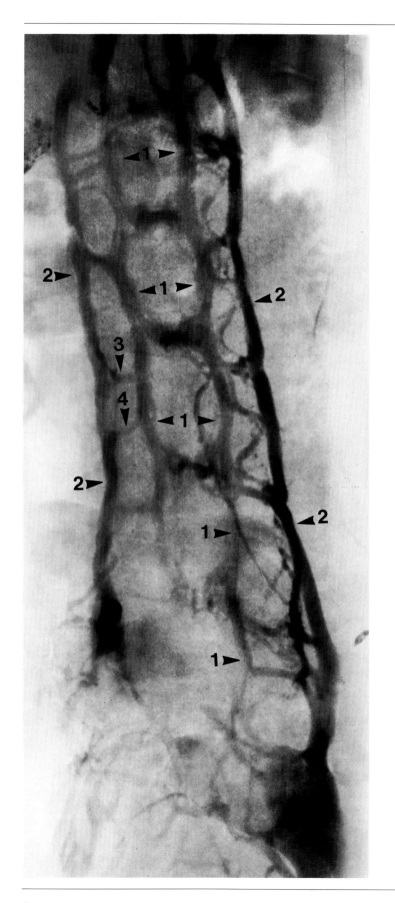

Figure 2

Effect of compression of the inferior vena cava during injection of contrast medium into the left common iliac vein. The dye goes entirely to the vertebral plexus, showing the epidural veins (*1*), the ascending lumbar veins (*2*), the superior (*3*) and inferior (*4*) veins of the lateral foramen

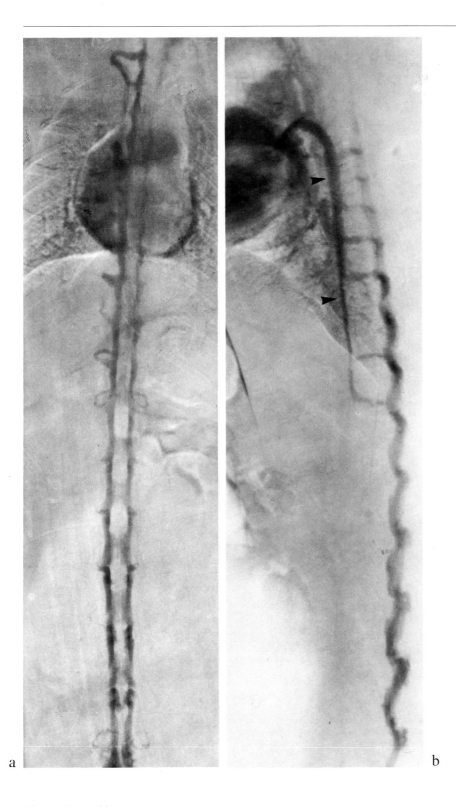

a

b

Figure 3 a and b

The same compression in a monkey during the injection of 3 ml contrast medium. The vertebral plexus is seen up to the dorsal and cervical levels. In (*b*), the azygos vein *(arrowheads)* is seen on a lateral view without the overlap of the vertebral plexus

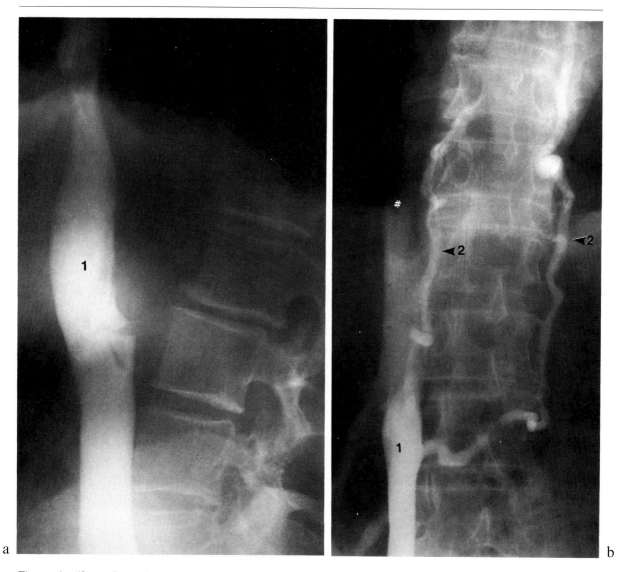

Figure 4a (lateral view) and b (AP view)

a Injection of contrast medium into the inferior vena cava gives optimal opacification of this vessel (*1*)

b The same injection repeated during a Valsalva maneuver. The vena cava is incompletely outlined (*1*) and there is the appearance of a blockage at the level of the diaphragm (*#*), while the meningorachidian plexus is partly shown with its ascending lumbar veins (*2*)

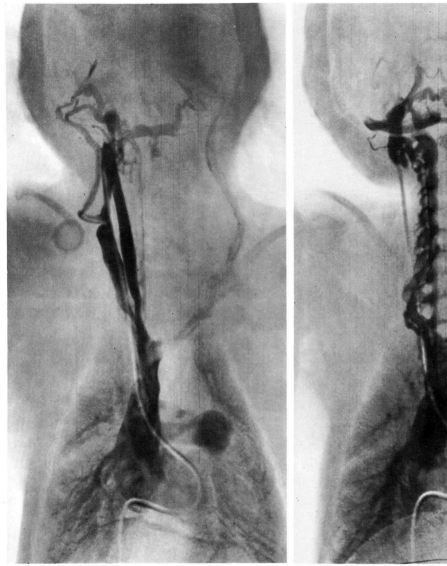

a

b

Figure 5a and b

a Injection in the monkey in the decubitus position of 2.5 cc Conray into the upper part of the right internal jugular vein shows the jugular veins on the right side

b The same injection is repeated after compression of the right internal jugular vein below the point of entry of the catheter. The cervical vertebral plexus is shown in detail, down to the superior vena cava

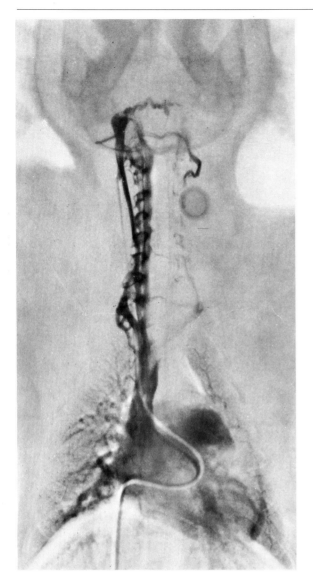

Figure 5 c

The same injection without compression but with the animal standing. Contrast medium again appears in the vertebral plexus, on the same side as the injection, while the internal and external jugular veins are not demonstrated

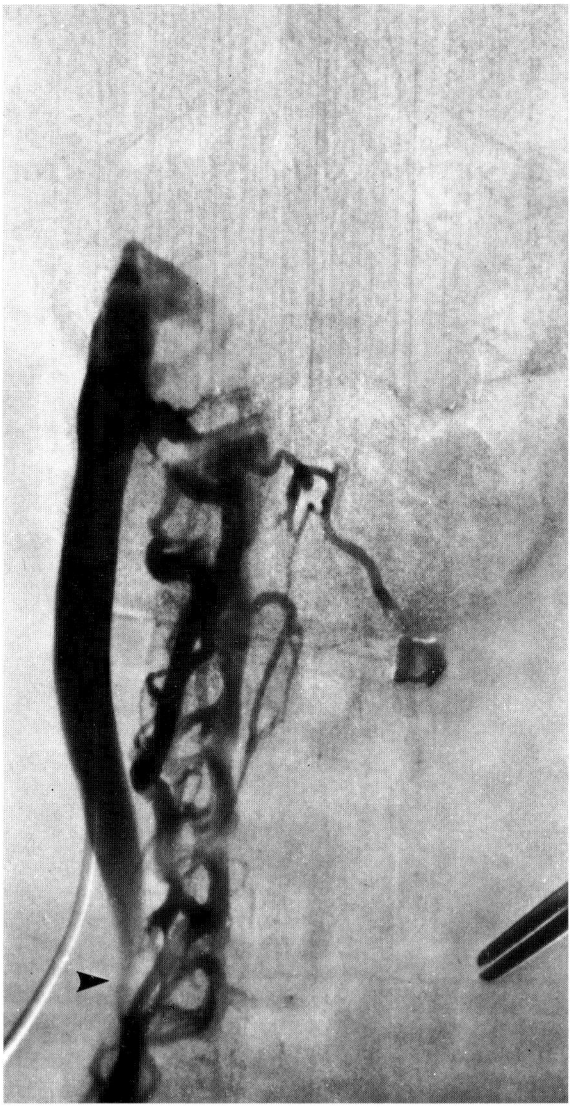

Figure 6

Injection of 8 cc Conray in the upper part of the internal jugular vein in man, with compression *(arrowhead)* below the site of the puncture. The contrast medium goes largely to the homolateral vertebral plexus, showing the paravertebral as well as epidural veins

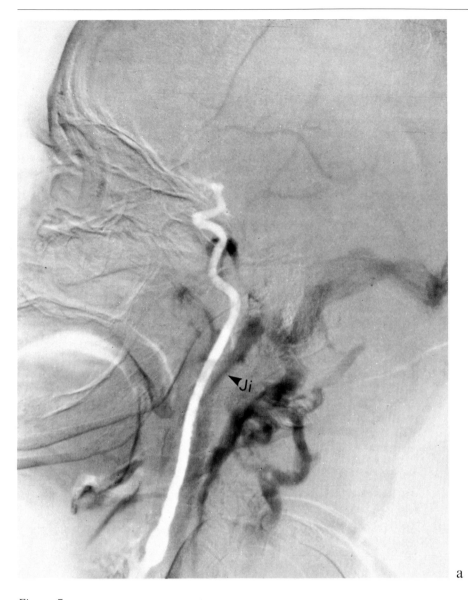

a

Figure 7a–c

Opacification of the cervical part of the meningorachidian plexus in the course of routine cerebral angiography

a The plexus and the jugular vein (*Ji*) are both seen
b The internal jugular vein is not seen but the plexus is filled, as well as the pterygoid veins (*Pp*) which drain into the external jugular vein (*Je*)
c The cervical meningorachidian plexus is also seen over a major part of its intravertebral course and at that particular time at least, seems to be the exclusive pathway of cerebral venous return

Small arrowheads point to the epidural portion of the plexus

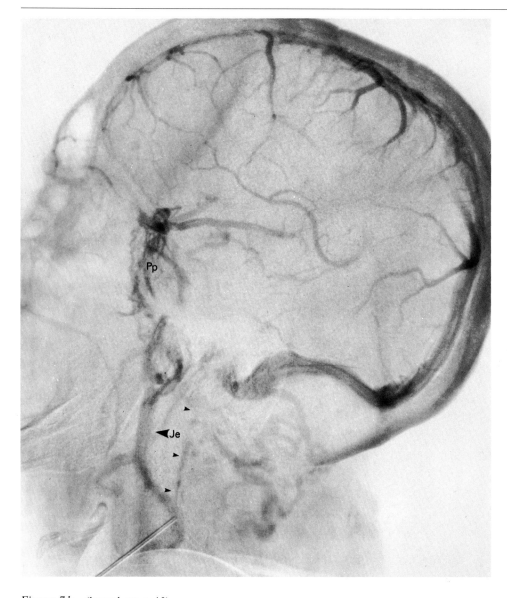

Figure 7b   (legend see p. 13)

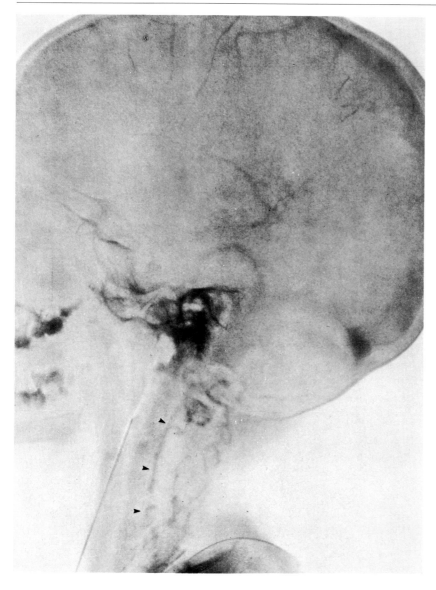

Figure 7c (legend see p. 13)

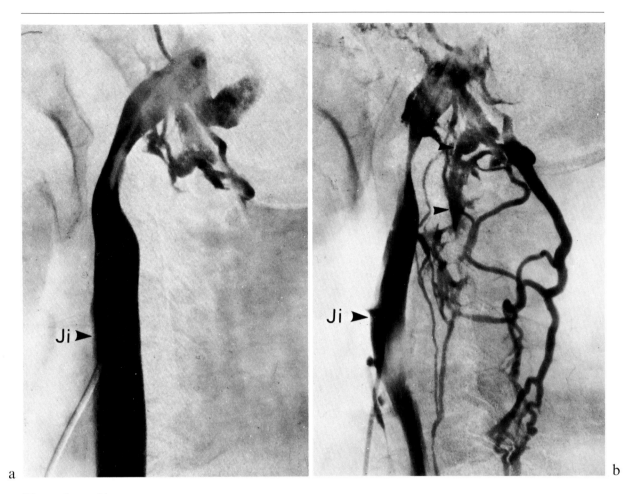

a

b

Figure 8 a and b

Injection in man of 10 cc Conray into the upper part of the internal jugular vein, without compression, in the decubitus position (a) and in the standing position (b). In (b), the internal jugular vein is definitely less well opacified and appears to be partly collapsed, while the paravertebral and epidural veins (*arrowheads*) are well shown. *Ji*, internal jugular vein

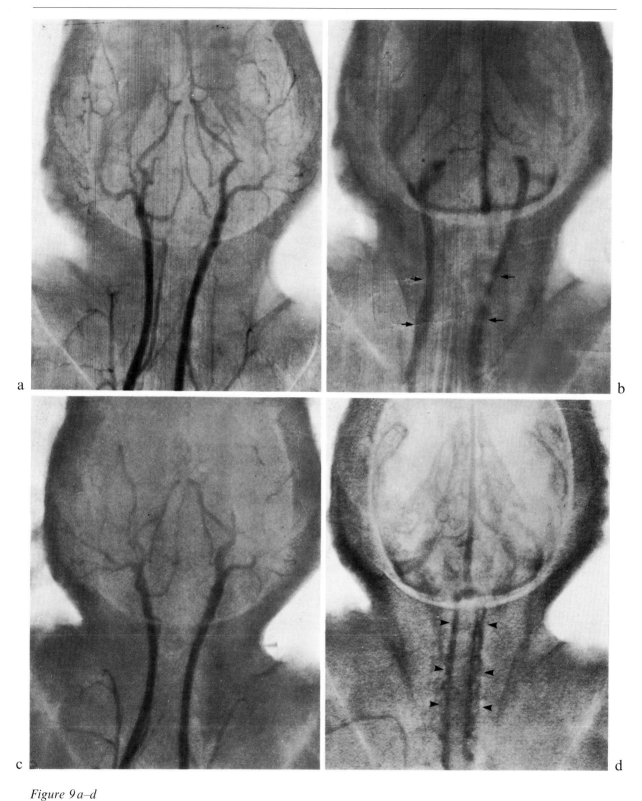

a

b

c

d

Figure 9 a–d

Arteriography by injection of contrast medium into the aortic arch of the monkey. The carotid and vertebral arteries are well seen in the decubitus (a) and standing (c) positions. Cerebral venous return takes place exclusively through the internal jugular veins *(arrows)* in the decubitus position (b) and takes place through the vertebral plexus *(arrowheads)* in the standing position (d)

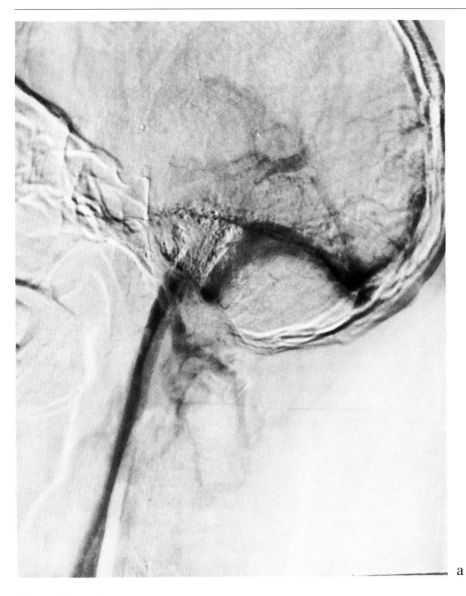

a

Figure 10 a and b

Effect of body position on the venous phase of vertebral arteriography (human). In the decubitus position venous drainage takes place almost exclusively through the jugular veins, which are well opacified (a). In the standing position, cerebral venous return takes place preferentially through the vertebral plexus (b), and the jugular veins are less well opacified

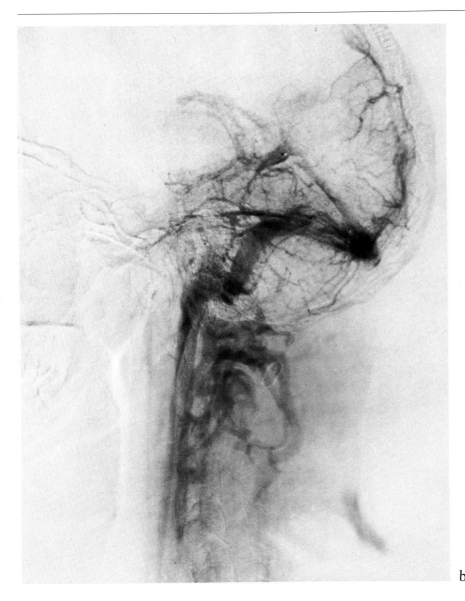

b

Figure 10b

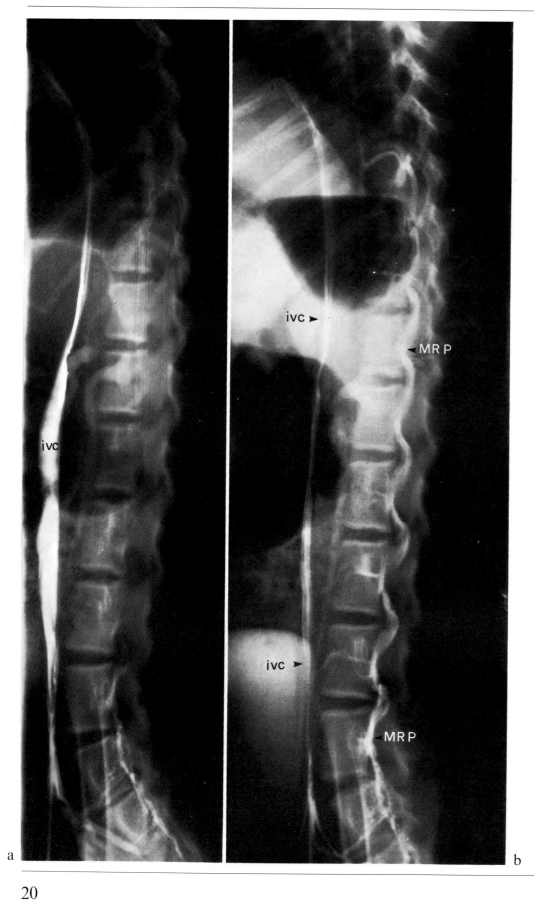

a

b

Figure
11 a and b

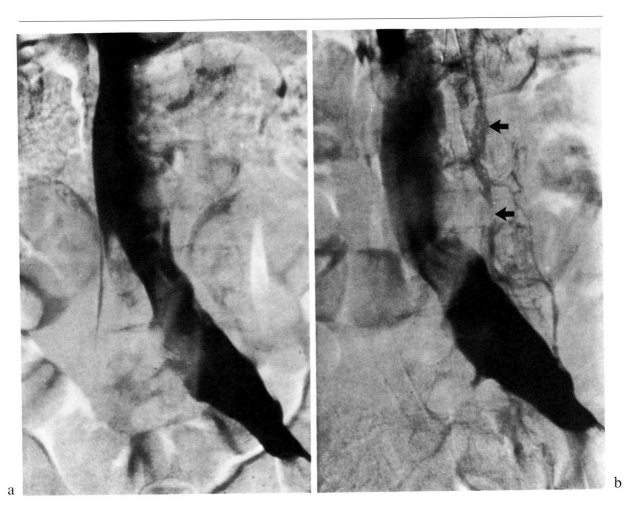

a   b

Figure 12a and b

Injection of contrast medium into the left iliac vein of
man in the horizontal (a) and the vertical positions with
the head down (b). (Courtesy of Dr. THERON.) In (b)
the contrast medium passes into the MRP, which appears
well opacified, particularly in its intrarachidian course
(arrows)

◁ *Figure 11a and b*

Injection of the contrast medium at the origin of the
inferior vena cava of the monkey. Lateral projections

a Horizontal position. Although a small quantity of contrast medium flows back into the anastomotic branches
of the MRP, the vena cava seems to be the exclusive
pathway of venous return

b Inverted position. Same injection with the animal vertical and the head down. The contrast medium now
passes preferentially in the MRP, which is well opacified
up to the azygos vein. The inferior vena cava is thinner
and appears to be partially collapsed

ivc Inferior vena cava; *MRP* Meningorachidian plexus

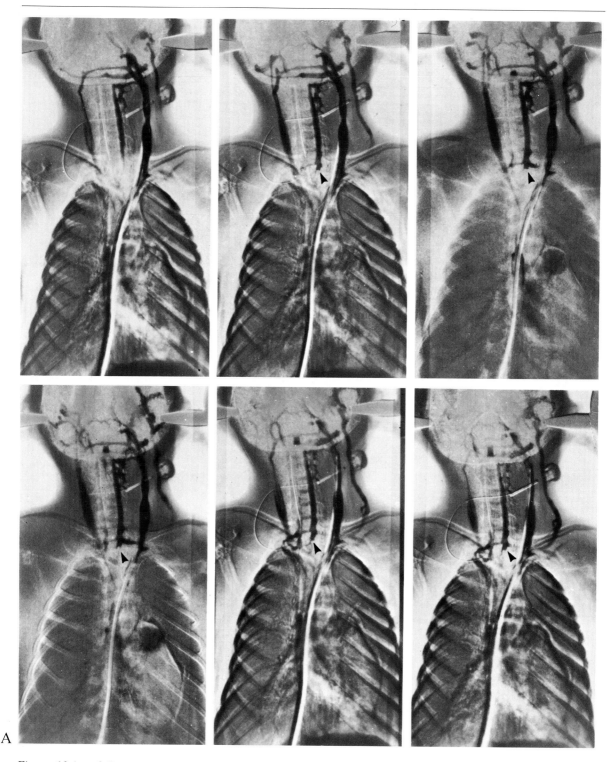

A

Figure 13A and B

Injection of 2.5 cc Conray into the internal jugular vein of a monkey subjected to high intrathoracic pressure. In (A), the injection is performed in the decubitus position.

The jugular veins appear to be distended as the entrance of the blood into the chest cavity is blocked. The vertebral plexus is not seen below C7 *(arrowhead)*. In (B), a similar

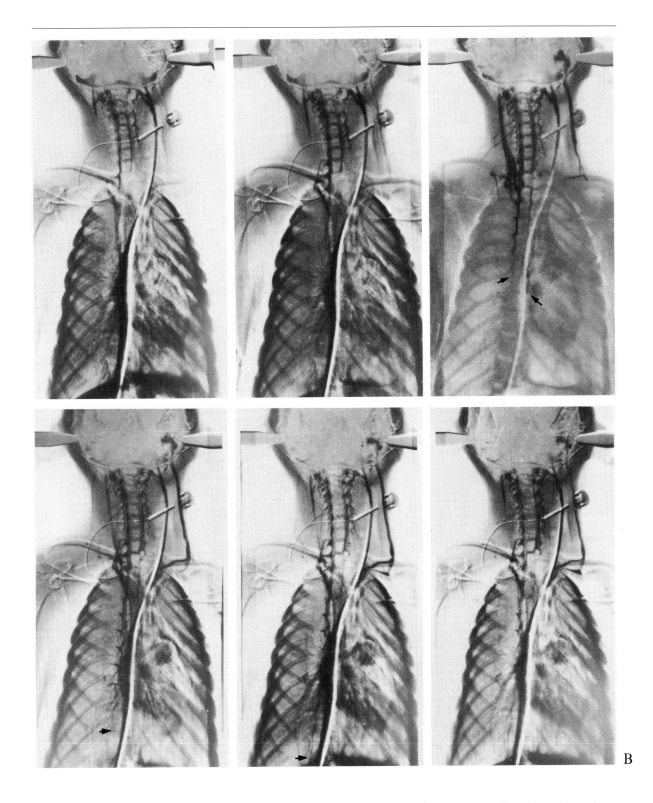

B

injection in the upright position does not fill the jugular veins to the same extent but the vertebral plexus is better opacified down to the level of the heart *(arrows)*. The upright position thus appears to allow the vertebral plexus to function as an outlet of overflow when high intrathoracic pressure interferes with venous return

Chapter 2

Lumbar Phlebography

2.1. Anatomic Radiology

J. Théron and J. Moret

Accurate radiologic description of the lumbar epidural veins has been slowed down by technical difficulties and an anatomic error. For precise anatomic analysis of the lumbar epidural veins, they must be well opacified along the complete length of the lumbosacral spinal canal. Injection into the ascending lumbar vein does not always ensure good filling of the epidural veins in front of the L5–S1 intervertebral disc: The origin of the ascending lumbar vein is located in front of or above this disc so the contrast medium is often carried along by the normal ascending venous flow. This led to errors of interpretation and consequently prevented the spread of the technique. Catheterization of the lateral sacral veins (see Sect 2.2) circumvented this problem in permitting, when associated with compression of the inferior vena cava, a nonphysiologic but complete opacification of the lumbosacral veins (Fig. 14).

The anatomic error was in fact a wrong interpretation of the original works by Breschet [11] that led to the description in radiologic publications of two anterior and two posterior longitudinal epidural veins. However, some authors who performed lateral projections in phlebography (see figure of the Foreword and Fig. 45, Sect. 2.3, and Fig. 55, Sect. 2.4), presumed that the posterior veins were small because they could not see them on this projection. Acutally, this anatomic conception did not fit with the results of the pathologic phlebograms and led to errors in interpretation, which caused the technique to be considered unreliable.

In 1975, we mentioned that our phlebograms suggested that the four longitudinal veins were anterior and located in the anterolateral angles of the spinal canal (Fig. 15). This hypothesis was confirmed by the anatomic work of Larde [54] and Renard et al. [70].

Contrary to the extravertebral venous system, the epidural veins have a very constant morphologic pattern. They usually present as two thick symmetrical venous strips, the morphology of which is identical in front of each intervertebral disc down to L5–S1 (Fig. 16 and 17). The venous strip deviates laterally in front of each intervertebral disc and then medially in front of the middle of each vertebral body where it unites with the contralateral homolog forming a dense retrocoporeal plexus hugging the medial side of the vertebral pedicle. This plexus is anterior to the posterior longitudinal ligament but in front of the disc the epidural veins are posterior to the ligament (Fig. 18). It is often difficult to differentiate the medial from the lateral epidural veins but this distinction is sometimes possible (Fig. 17).

In front of L5–S1 the appearance of the epidural veins is different; the lateral epidural vein deviates more laterally and the medial vein more medially close to the midline. A characteristic group of four veins is then recognizable, the integrity of which is essential to rule out a lesion of the L5–S1 intervertebral disc. At this level and at the levels where the medial vein can be recognized, it appears markedly more tortuous than the lateral one. Phlebography is a particularly reliable technique in front of L5–S1, because of the increased thickness of the epidural space at this level, which leeds to rather frequent false negative results on radiculography.

Epidural veins of the respective sides are symmetrical to each other side; this symmetry represents a major point in the interpretation of a phlebogram, particularly in front of L5–S1. The epidural veins have constant relationships with the intervertebral discs, as opposed to the nerve roots, the emergence and course of which are quite varied (Fig. 19).

Epidural veins are connected at each disc level to the extravertebral system by the veins of the lateral foramen. A superior and an inferior vein can be schematically recognized (Fig. 16). In fact the veins of the lateral foramen are frequently multiple (Fig. 17) and do not have the constant appearance of the epidural veins. Absence of opacification in front of one disc level will be considered pathologic only if the corresponding veins of the superior and inferior levels are normally opacified. The morphology of the ascending lumbar veins is also quite varied. On the left side this vein is usually of good caliber and can be a single or a plexiform vein; it arises from the common iliac vein but can also arise from the internal iliac vein. On the right side, this vein frequently has a smaller caliber and may arise from a common stem with an iliac vein.

Epidural veins are connected inferiorly with the lateral sacral veins. There are usually two main lateral sacral veins on each side that arise from the internal iliac vein but sometimes from the common iliac vein; the internal iliac vein may be single or double and the angiographer should adapt his technique to the variations which are, here again, quite frequent.

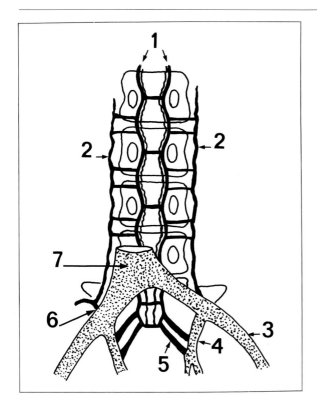

Figure 14

The anatomic relationships of the lumbar epidural veins with the extravertebral veins

1 Epidural veins
2 Ascending lumbar veins
3 External iliac vein
4 Internal iliac vein
5 Lateral sacral veins
6 Common stem between an iliac vein and the right ascending lumbar vein
7 Inferior vena cava

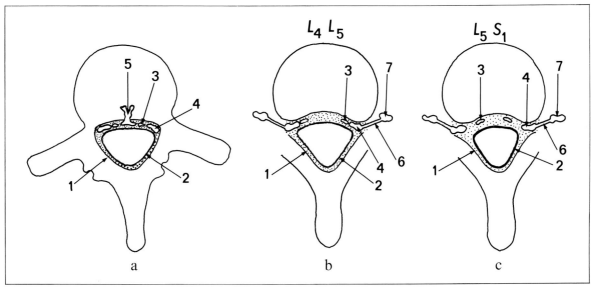

Figure 15 a–c

The anatomic relationships of the epidural veins with the intervertebral discs and vertebral bodies

a Section passing through a lumbar vertebral body
b Section passing through the intervertebral disc L4–L5
c Same section passing through L5–S1

1 Epidural space
2 Dura mater
3 Medial epidural vein
4 Lateral epidural vein
5 Basivertebral vein
6 Veins of the lateral foramen
7 Ascending lumbar vein

Note that there is no posterior longitudinal epidural vein. Note also the juxtaposition of the medial and lateral epidural veins, at each discal level, down to L5–S1 where they spread apart and can be differentiated on a phlebogram. In front of each vertebral body the medial and lateral veins become closer to the contralateral veins and receive the basivertebral vein; together they form the venous retrocorporeal anastomosis

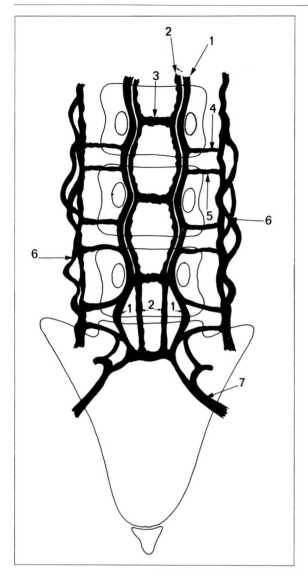

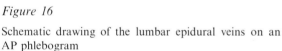

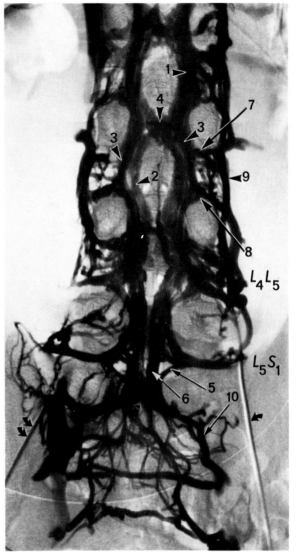

Figure 16

Schematic drawing of the lumbar epidural veins on an AP phlebogram

1 Lateral epidural vein. *2* Medial epidural vein; this vein is more tortuous than the lateral one, from which it usually cannot be distinguished down to L5–S1 where they spread apart. *3* Retrocorporeal anastomosis that also receives the basivertebral vein. *4* Superior vein of the lateral foramen. *5* Inferior vein of the lateral foramen. These veins of the lateral foramen are sometimes more numerous. *6* Ascending lumbar vein. *7* Lateral sacral vein

Figure 17

Normal AP lumbar phlebogram performed by catheterization of the left ascending lumbar vein *(arrow)* and of a right lateral sacral vein *(double arrow)*

1 Usual pattern of the epidural veins down to L5–S1; the medial and the lateral cannot usually be differentiated. *2* In this case at L3–L4, the medial epidural vein can be recognized. *3* Lateral epidural vein. *4* Retrocorporeal venous anastomosis between the right and left epidural longitudinal veins; this anastomosis receives the blood flow of the basivertebral vein. *5* Lateral epidural vein at L5–S1. *6* Medial epidural vein nearing the midline at L5–S1. *7* Superior vein of the left L3–L4 lateral foramen. *8* Inferior vein of the lateral foramen. Note the different pattern of the veins of the left L4–L5 lateral foramen where they present as a plexus. *9* Ascending lumbar vein that may be double or plexiform. *10* Lateral sacral vein

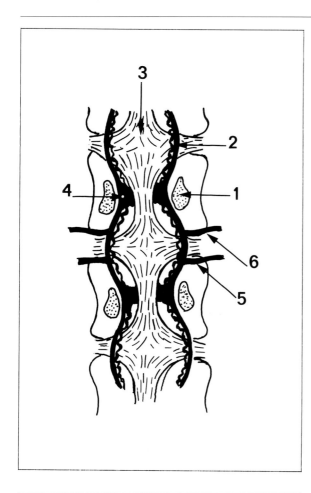

Figure 18

Schematic drawing of the relationships of the epidural veins to the intervertebral disc and posterior longitudinal ligament. The veins are seen from behind after removal of the posterior arch of the spinal canal

1 Pedicle
2 Epidural veins in front of an intervertebral disc; they are situated behind the posterior longitudinal ligament
3 The posterior longitudinal ligament is thicker on the midline in front of the intervertebral disc
4 Retrocorporeal venous anastomosis that receives the basivertebral vein; the posterior longitudinal ligament is now behind the veins
5 Inferior vein of the lateral foramen
6 Superior vein of the lateral foramen

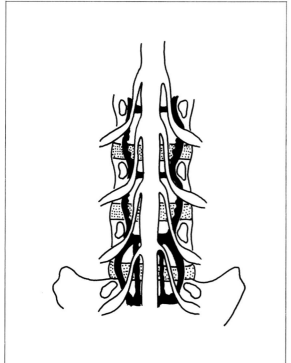

Figure 19

Schematic drawing of the anatomic relationships of the lumbar nerve roots to the vertebral bodies, the intervertebral disc, and the epidural veins. The constant relationships of the epidural veins to the vertebral bodies and the intervertebral discs contrast with the rather frequent variations of emergence of the nerve roots from the dural sac. Usually each nerve root emerges from the anterior part of the dural sac in front of the vertebral body situated above the lateral foramen from which they leave the spinal canal. Conversely, each nerve root crosses the disc that is situated under the vertebral body in front of which they emerge from the dural sac

2.2. Technique, Pitfalls, Complications

J. Moret and J. Théron

The patient is sedated half an hour before the procedure (Tranxene–atropine). Phlebography is performed under local anesthesia via a bilateral venous femoral approach in strict sterile conditions. The catheters are introduced into the femoral veins using the Seldinger technique. To prevent venous thrombosis as a result of the procedure, 30–50 mg heparin is injected into one of the veins as soon as the catheters are in place.

The catheters are 60 cm long and 5 F in caliber tapered on 32 or 35 guide wire. Their tip is shaped with a more or less compound curve (Fig. 20). Lumbar phlebography needs experience to be regularly successful and the angiographer should adapt his technique to the particular extravertebral system in each case.

In most cases good opacification of the epidural veins is obtained by injection into two extravertebral veins: an ascending lumbar vein and a lateral sacral vein. The left ascending lumbar vein is the more frequently chosen because of its larger diameter; the catheter is positioned in front of the veins of the left lateral foramen L5–S1 for the most satisfactory filling. A right or left lateral sacral vein is injected depending on which is easier to catheterize; midline anastomosis usually permits equally good opacification of the epidural veins when a right or left sacral vein is chosen. Various technical modalities are showed on Figures 21, 22, and 23.

An angiography series (1 film/s for 10 s) is performed during injection of 20 cc of contrast medium (Telebrix 30 not yet available in the United Kingdom or the United States) on each side at a rate of 3 cc/s. Immediately before injection an abdominal compression is set with a balloon to compress the vena cava and force the contrast medium to enter the epidural veins; the patient may also be asked to perform a Valsalva maneuver during the series to improve even further the preferential filling of the intraspinal veins. A complementary series without abdominal compression (see Sect. 2.4) or in the upright position (see Sect. 2.8) is sometimes performed in special cases.

Only an AP projection is usually necessary and one series is sufficient in most cases. When the veins situated in front of L5–S1 are not sufficiently opacified, a second series is performed after catheterization of a lateral sacral vein on each side (Figs. 24 and 25). Subtractions are systematically performed after the procedure, before interpretation.

In a few cases (about 2%) the epidural veins are poorly opacified by injection into a lateral sacral and an ascending lumbar vein. This is usually due to anatomic variations of the lateral sacral veins. In this case, catheterization of a lumbar vein (L2 on the right or L3 on the left) is performed and injection into this vein coupled with injection into an ascending lumbar vein usually assures far better opacification of the epidural veins (Figs. 26a, b and 27a, b). These lumbar veins studied by C. Gillot and B. Singer [44] seem to have special anatomic connections with the venous epidural system (Fig. 28a, b).

2.2.1. Pitfalls

All pitfalls are related to technical problems when the extravertebral veins chosen for injection do not provide correct opacification of the epidural veins along the complete length of the lumbosacral canal (Fig. 29). It is absolutely necessary in order to ascertain a pathologic venous interrruption, that the superior and inferior limits of the compression are well visualized.

2.2.2. Complications

Venous extravasations can occur in the course of the procedure; their frequency depends mainly on the angiographer's experience and almost never occur once he or she is skilled. The patient experiences a localized pain in the area of the extravasation that disappears rapidly and never has any secondary consequences. After a few minutes, the angiographer can proceed to catheterize another extravertebral vein.

Venous thrombosis of the inferior limb with eventual pulmonary embolus can also occur after the procedure as a complication of venous catheterization. The few cases observed occurred after surgery and represented less than 1% of the cases out of approximately 1 500 procedures. Their incidence is now even lower with the systematic use of heparin during the procedure. For the same reason, we also prefer using a technique other than phlebography in the work-up of patients with a history of thrombophlebitis. When surgery is decided upon, the patient is routinely administered anti-inflammatory drugs (phenylbutazone); phlebography presumably predisposes to thrombophlebitis when associated with surgery, particularly in those patients who remain in bed, sometimes for several weeks, because of sciatica.

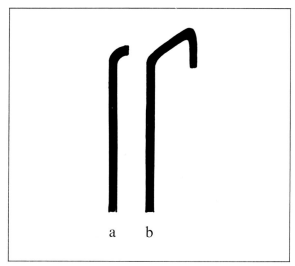

Figure 20 a and b

Tips of the catheters used to perform lumbar phlebography

a Plain curve

b Compound curve that facilitates the crossing of the catheter from an iliac vein on one side toward the internal iliac vein on the other side to opacify a lateral sacral vein

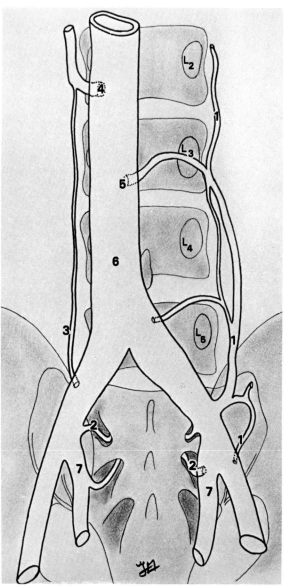

Figure 21

Schematic drawing of the various extravertebral veins, catheterization of which permits the opacification of the epidural veins

1 Left ascending lumbar vein
2 Lateral sacral veins
3 Right ascending lumbar vein not present in all cases
4 Second right lumbar vein
5 Third left lumbar vein
6 Inferior vena cava
7 Internal iliac vein

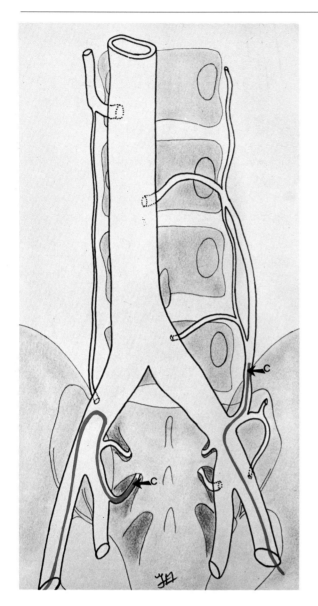

Figure 22

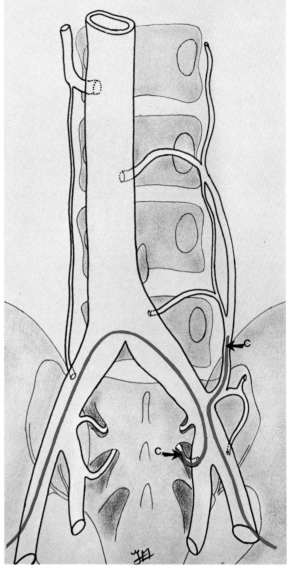

Figure 23

Figures 22 and 23

The various modes of catheterization of the left ascending
lumbar vein and of a lateral sacral vein. *C* Catheter

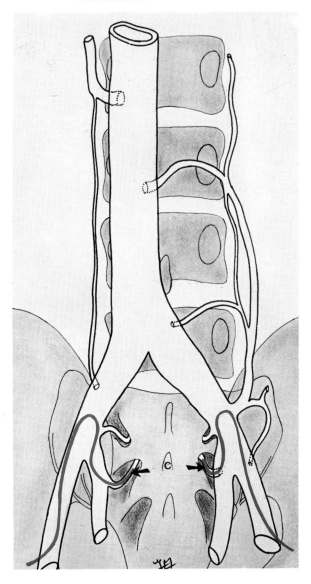

Figure 24

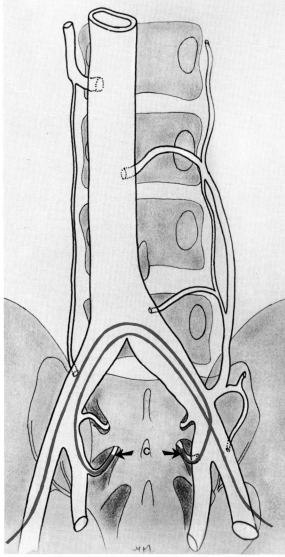

Figure 25

Figures 24 and 25

The various technical possibilities for bilateral catheterization of a lateral sacral vein. *C* Catheter

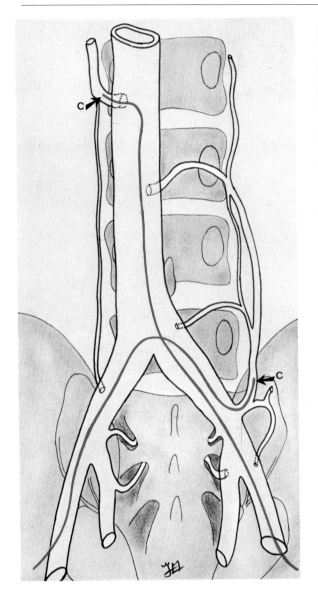

Figure 26 a

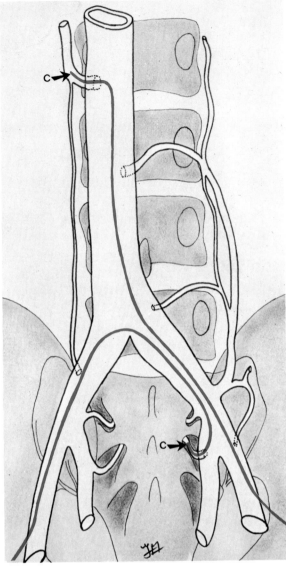

Figure 26 b

Figure 26 a and b

Various modes of catheterization of a left ascending lumbar vein or a lateral sacral vein associated with catheterization of the second right lumbar vein

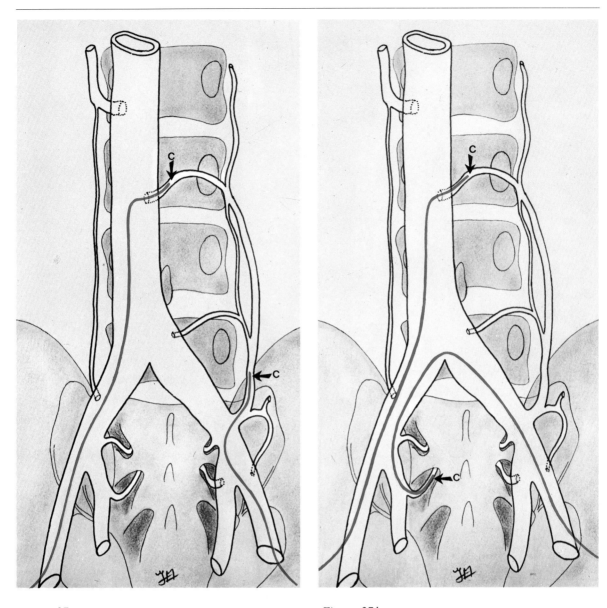

Figure 27a

Figure 27b

Figure 27a and b
Techniques using the third left lumbar vein

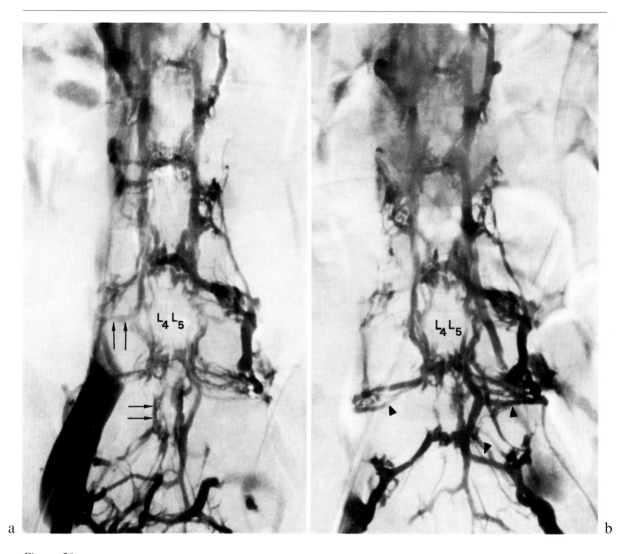

a   b

Figure 28

a Spinal phlebography performed by injection of the left
 ascending lumbar vein and of a right lateral sacral vein
b Same patient. Injection of the left ascending lumbar
 vein and of the second right lumbar vein.
The *double arrows* indicate the veins opacified on (a) and
not seen on (b)

The *arrowheads* indicate the veins opacified on (b) and
not seen on (a)

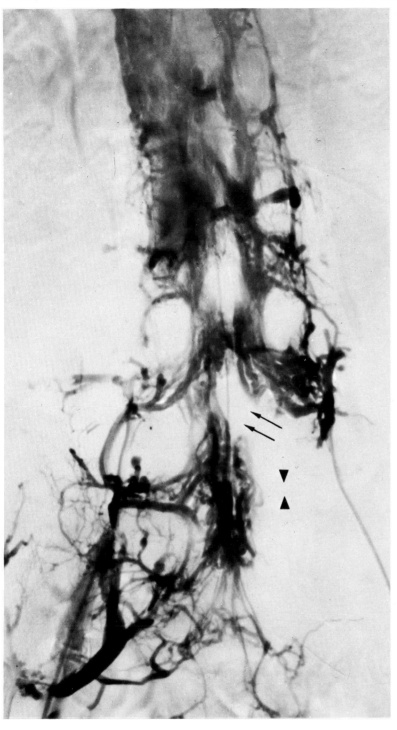

a

Figure 29a

Spinal phlebography performed by injection of the left ascending lumbar and right lateral sacral veins. The epidural veins are not opacified on the left in front of L4–L5 disc level *(double arrow)*. The veins of the left lateral foramen L5–S1 are not opacified either *(arrowheads)*

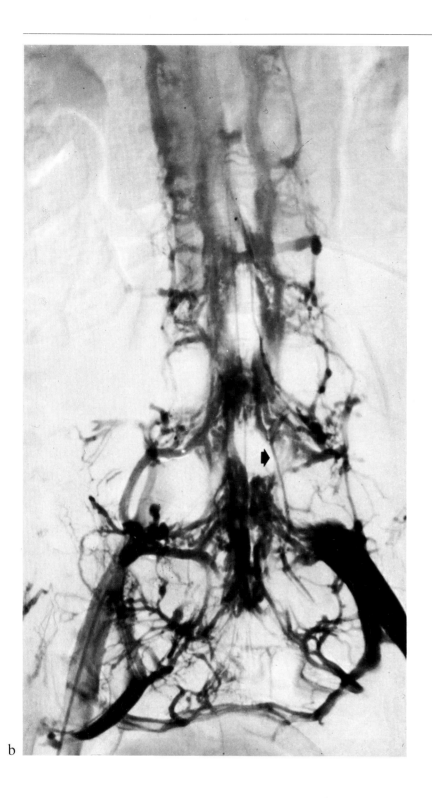

b

Figure 29b

Same patient. Injection of a lateral sacral vein on both sides. On this injection, only an interruption of the left medial epidural vein and a displacement of the lateral epidural vein persist, indicating the exact localization of the disc herniation *(arrow)*

2.3. Disc Herniations

J. Théron, J. Moret and J. Vignaud

Epidural veins represent an important anatomic landmark in the diagnosis of disc herniations because they are located in the anterolateral angles of the spinal canal in contact with the intervertebral disc. Any disc lesion that compresses a nerve root will previously compress the corresponding epidural veins interposed between the disc and the nerve root.

Accurate diagnosis can be made only if good opacification of the epidural veins is obtained along the complete length of the lumbosacral canal; as seen in Section 2.2, this is usually obtained by injection into an ascending lumbar vein and a lateral sacral vein with abdominal compression that forces the contrast medium into the intravertebral veins. When the epidural veins appear interrupted it is necessary to visualize the superior and inferior limits of compression to be sure that this nonopacification is not due to technical inadequacies.

An AP projection is usually sufficient; lateral projection is rarely used because of the superimposition of the right and left epidural veins, which does not permit an accurate study of a unilateral compression. A series without compression is sometimes performed to make minor compressions more obvious (see Sect. 2.4). When opacification of epidural veins is technically satisfactory, phlebographic diagnosis of disc herniation is easy in most cases; the basic sign is the localized interruption of the epidural veins. In our experience the most frequent phlebographic signs are as follows:

1. Complete interruption of the venous longitudinal strip on one side or on both sides in front of the pathologic intervertebral disc (Figs. 30–34). Epidural veins frequently present a tapered pattern before the interruption (Fig. 31) due to compression of the lumen of the vein by the disc herniation (see Sect. 2.5). When venous compression is less marked it is sometimes possible to obtain faint opacification of the compressed veins on the series with abdominal compression but in the series without compression these veins would appear totally interrupted (Fig. 45).

2. Selective interruption of the medial (Figs. 35, 36, 37) or the lateral (Figs. 38, 39–40) epidural vein is more easily demonstrated in front of L5–S1 where the veins spread apart. At most the disc herniation can determine a simple notch on the epidural venous strip (Figs. 41, 42).

3. Nonopacification of the veins of a lateral foramen in the case of lateral extension of disc material is a sign of value only when other veins of the lateral foramen on the same side are well opacified.

4. Dilatation of the epidural veins adjacent to the herniation due to the bypass of the obstacle by the venous blood flow (Fig. 43).

5. Dilatation of the retrocorporeal venous anastomoses situated above and below the pathologic disc (Figs. 38, 44, 45 b). This sign seems to visualize the so-called epidural varices that were thought to be responsible for some cases of sciatica.

Because the epidural veins are situated in the anterolateral angles of the spinal canal, the only type of disc herniation that could basically be overlooked on phlebography is the herniation arising strictly on the midline and consequently passing between the epidural veins. This could be true only above L5–S1 because at this level the medial epidural veins are situated closer to the midline and the disc can be completely investigated using phlebography. In fact, in most cases, even in front of the other discs, a midline herniation determines a modification, at least unilateral, of the epidural veins that calls for a complementary investigation such as a radiculography (Fig. 50). It seems also that a distinction can be drawn on phlebograms between the "true" disc herniation and the "nonpathologic" disc protrusion that corresponds to a simple bulging of the disc and may be observed in asymptomatic (or still asymptomatic) patients: On the phlebogram, in this latter case, a posterior regular displacement of the epidural veins without interruption is observed in front of the disc on lateral projection (Fig. 45).

Phlebography could be used as the first technique of investigation of disc herniations but, considering the great number of patients presenting with sciatica, and having to face the practical impossibility of performing phlebography on each of them, we often use radiculography as the first and frequently the only technique of investigation. If the radiculogram is significantly abnormal at the level indicated by the clinical symptoms, the patient is usually operated upon without phlebography. Conversely, when radiculography is negative or does not show sufficiently significant signs or when its results do not correlate with the clinical symptoms, phlebography is then performed. However, phlebography remains for us the first technique of investigation in two circumstances: [1] In cases of sciatica with palsy where it provides enough informations to operate on the patient in an emergency and consequently increases the possibilities of relieving the palsy. [2] In patients who cannot keep the upright position necessary for performing radiculography because of hyperalgic sciatica.

Phlebography can also be used for the investigation of postoperative recurrence of sciatica, but the local surgical coagulation of the epidural vein to control the bleeding makes the demonstration of a venous interruption value less at the operated disc level; on the other hand, a pathologic pattern of the veins situated superiorly, inferiorly, or contralaterally to the site of surgery has great diagnostic value (Fig. 46). However, the veins are not always interrupted after surgery (Fig. 47) and the demonstration of normal veins will permit a recurrence at the site of the operation to be ruled out (see also Sect. 2.7).

The advantages of phlebography as compared to radiculography in the work-up of disc herniations are:

1. Greater accuracy in the diagnosis of disc herniations arising laterally in the spinal canal at each disc level; in front of L5–S1, any kind of disc herniations is better visualized because of the thickness of the epidural space and the particular position of the epidural veins at this level (Fig. 44). This is especially so in cases of megadural sac (see Sect. 2.6).

2. The possibility of obtaining precise information on the discs situated above and below the herniation. This is important for decisions regarding preventive excision of the other pathologic discs demonstrated on phlebography to avoid postoperative recurrence due to the increased work-load on these discs if left in place after surgery (Figs. 48, 49) (see Sect. 2.5). The problem is identical when clinical symptomatology is unilateral and the phlebogram shows bilateral interruption of the veins; a bilateral surgical approach can then be discussed to perform a better disc excision and avoid a secondary migration of the contralateral pathologic disc material toward the cavity of the disc excision.

3. Greater accuracy in cases of arachnoiditis (see Sect. 2.7).

4. Excellent tolerance by the patient due to the absence of introduction of contrast me-

dium into the subarachnoid spaces and the performance of the procedure in the supine position.

The disadvantages are:

1. The theoretical possibility of overlooking a herniation strictly located on the midline at the disc levels above L5–S1 (Fig. 50).

2. The absence of specificity of the venous interruption and particularly the impossibility, on the phlebogram alone, of differentiating an anterior compression due to a disc from a posterior one due to intraspinal conditions such as a tumor

3. The longer time taken in the performance of the procedure

4. The risk of thromboembolic complications which, even if minimal, contraindicates this technique in patients with a history of thrombophlebitis.

5. The prerequisites: an experienced angiographer, a team of trained technicians, and angiographic equipment.

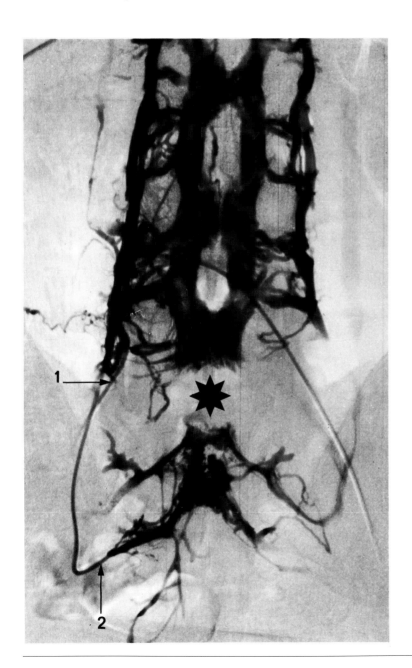

Figure 30

Bilateral L5–S1 disc herniation. Lumbar phlebography by catheterization of the right ascending lumbar vein (*1*) and of a right lateral sacral vein (*2*). Bilateral interruption of the epidural venous flow in front of the L5–S1 intervertebral disc *(star)*

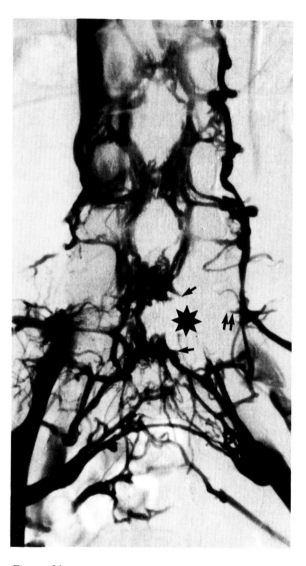

Figure 31

Left disc herniation L5–S1 *(star)*. Interruption of the left lateral and medial epidural veins in front of L5–S1 *(arrows)*. The interruption of the corresponding veins of the lateral foramen *(double arrow)* is due to extension of disc material into it

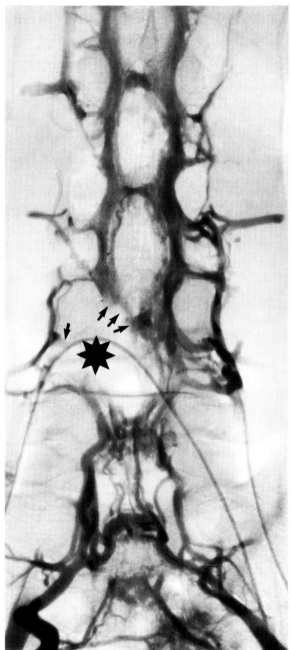

Figure 32

Right disc herniation L4–L5 *(star)*. Nonopacification of the right epidural veins with impression of the disc herniation on the superior part of the interruption *(arrows)*. Note the interruption of the superior vein of the corresponding lateral foramen *(vertical arrow)*

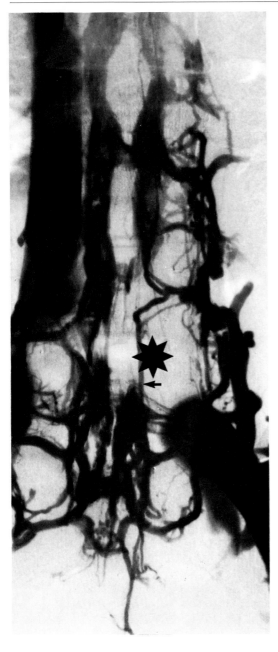

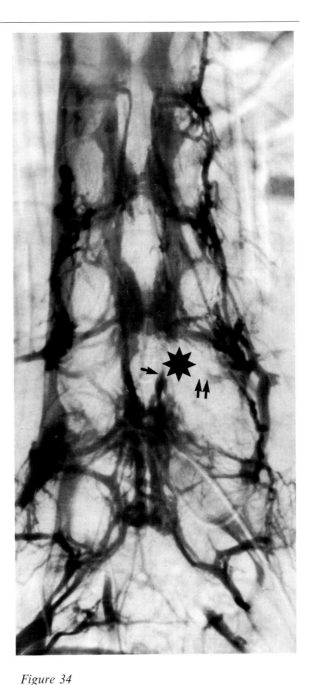

Figure 33

Left disc herniation L4–L5. Interruption of the epidural veins in front of the L4–L5 intervertebral disc on the left side *(star)*. Note the opacification of a dilated posterior vein *(arrow)* that should not be mistaken for a longitudinal anterior epidural vein

Figure 34

Left disc herniation L4–L5 with extension of disc material into the lateral foramen *(star)*. Note the interruption of the medial and lateral epidural veins in front of the L4–L5 intervertebral disc on the left side *(arrow)*. The inferior vein of the corresponding lateral foramen is also interrupted because of the extension of disc material into it *(double arrow)*

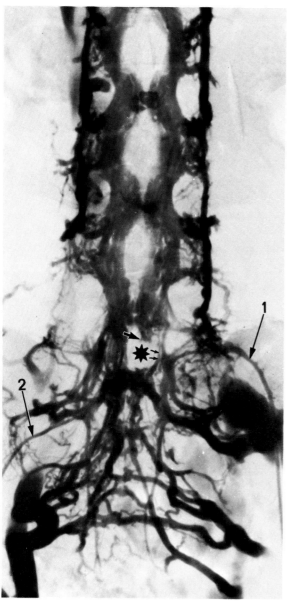

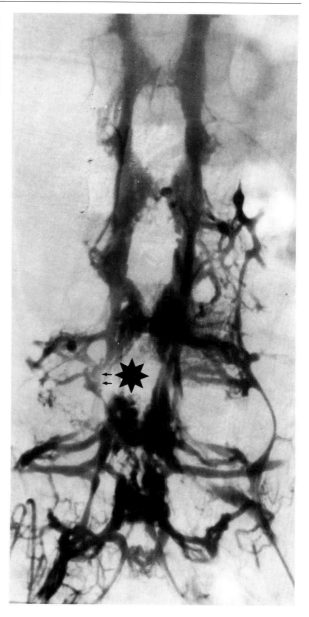

Figure 35

Spinal phlebography by catheterization of the left ascending lumbar (*1*) and of a right lateral sacral (*2*) veins. Left disc herniation L4–L5 *(star)*. Note the interruption of the left medial epidural vein in front of the L4–L5 intervertebral disc *(arrow)* with compression of the lateral epidural vein *(double arrow)*

Figure 36

Right disc herniation L4–L5 *(star)*. Note the compression and displacement of the lateral epidural vein *(double arrow)* and the interruption of the medial epidural vein

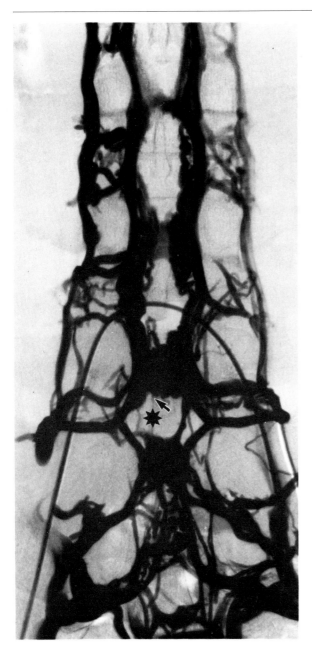

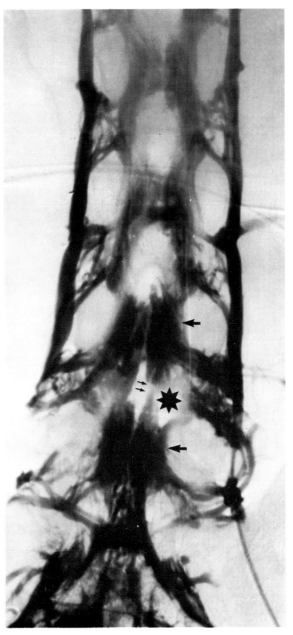

Figure 37

Medial right disc herniation L5–S1 *(star)*. Only the medial epidural vein is interrupted *(arrow)* because of the position of the disc lesion close to the midline. Normal pattern of the other veins

Figure 38

Left disc herniation L4–L5 *(star)*. Interruption of the lateral epidural vein with tapering of the medial epidural vein *(double arrow)*. Note the enhancement of the contrast medium in the dilated retrocorporeal anastomosis above and below the disc herniation *(arrows)*

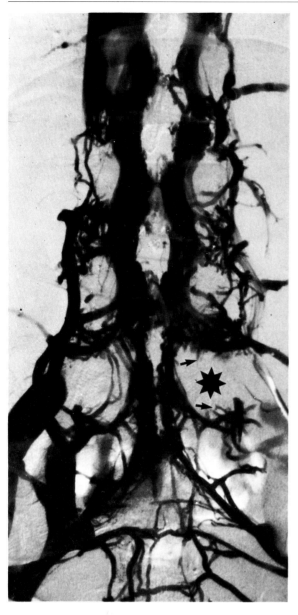

Figure 39

Left disc herniation L5–S1 (star). Interruption of the lateral epidural vein in front of the L5–S1 intervertebral disc on the left side *(arrows)*. Normal pattern of the medial epidural vein on the same side

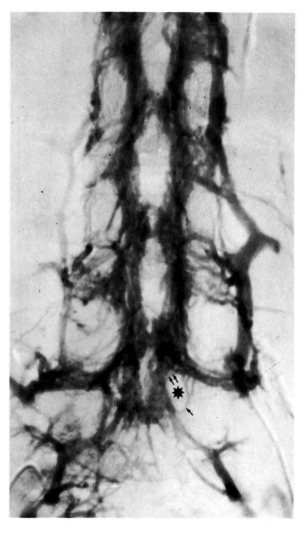

Figure 40

Left disc herniation L5–S1 *(star)*. Note the reduced caliber of the lateral epidural veins, appreciated by comparison with the opposite side, in front of L5–S1 on the left side. The medial epidural vein is also slightly displaced medially and presents a notch on its lateral side *(double arrow)*

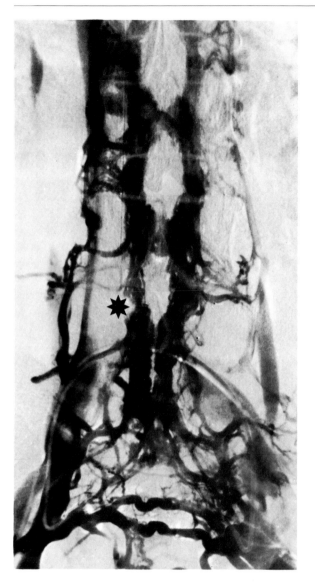

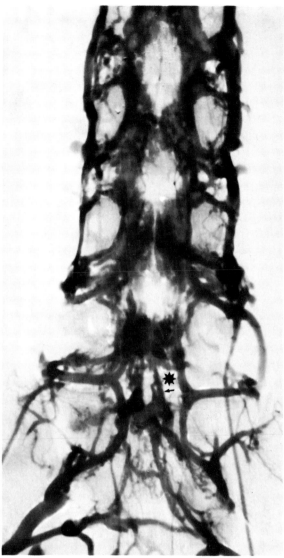

Figure 41

Lateral right disc herniation L4–L5 *(star)*. Partial interruption of the venous epidural strip on its lateral side by the disc lesion

Figure 42

Left disc herniation L5–S1 *(star)*. Partial interruption of the left medial epidural vein in front of L5–S1 with stretching of the remaining vein *(arrow)*

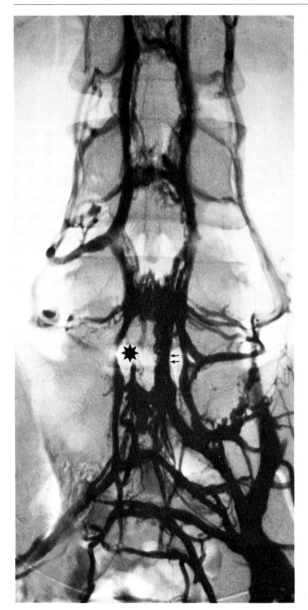

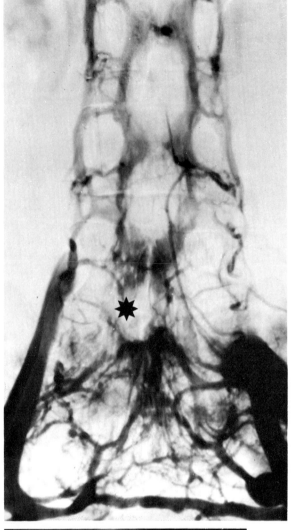

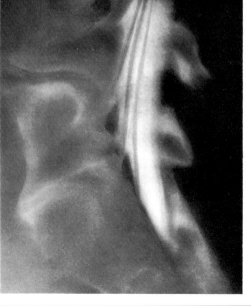

Figure 43

Right disc herniation L5–S1 *(star)*. On the right side, compression of the epidural veins, which are not completely interrupted. Dilatation of the left medial epidural vein secondary to the bypass of the disc lesion by the venous flow *(double arrow)*

Figure 44a and b   ▷

Right disc herniation L5–S1 *(star)*

a Lumbar phlebogram. Interruption of the right epidural veins in front of L5–S1 with dilatation of the venous anastomosis in front of S1
b Radiculogram (dimer X) using the tomographic technique shows a normal pattern of the nerve roots on the right side

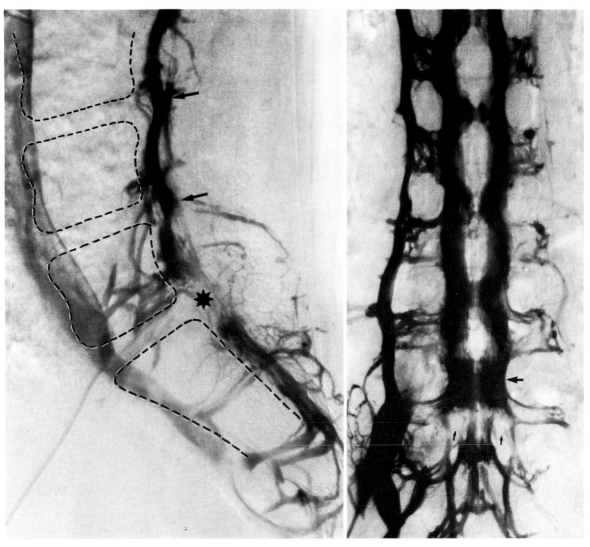

a

b

Figure 45 a and b

Bilateral disc herniation L5–S1

a Phlebography without compression of the inferior vena cava. Lateral projection. Interruption of the epidural veins in front of L5–S1 *(star)*. Note also the regular posterior displacement of the epidural veins in front of the superior discs *(arrows)* that could illustrate the difference between a "nonpathologic protrusion" and a disc herniation

b Same procedure. AP projection with compression of the inferior vena cava. The lateral epidural veins are interrupted in front of L5–S1 *(arrows)*. The retrocorporeal venous anastomosis situated in front of L5, above the disc herniation, appears dilated *(horizontal, arrow)*. The protrusions described on the lateral projection do not modify the veins on the AP projection.

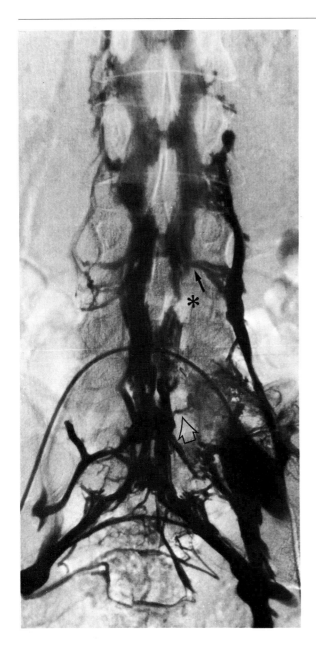

Figure 46

Disc excision L5–S1 for a left discal herniation four years previously. Presently left sciatic neuralgia L5. On phlebography is observed an interruption of lateral epidural vein in front of L5–S1 *(open arrow)*. This interruption cannot be interpreted as pathological since the patient has been operated on at this level. Conversely partial interruption of epidural veins in front of L4–L5 is significant and due to an other disc herniation *(star)*. Extension of disc material in the lateral foramen is proven by upper displacement of the medial portion of the inferior vein of the corresponding lateral foramen *(arrow)*

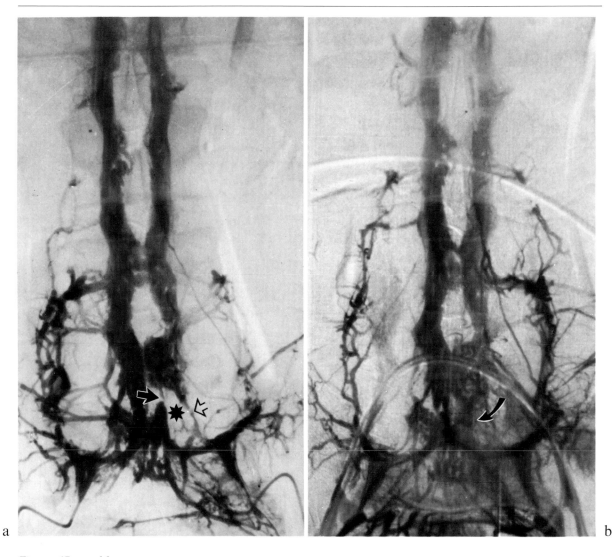

a   b

Figure 47a and b

a Left disc herniation L5–S1 *(star)* with interruption of the left medial epidural vein *(solid arrow)* and lateral displacement of the left lateral epidural vein *(open arrow)*

b Lumbar phlebography performed on the same patient after disc excision L5–S1. Note the opacification of the left medial epidural vein which was interrupted in (a) *(curved arrow)*

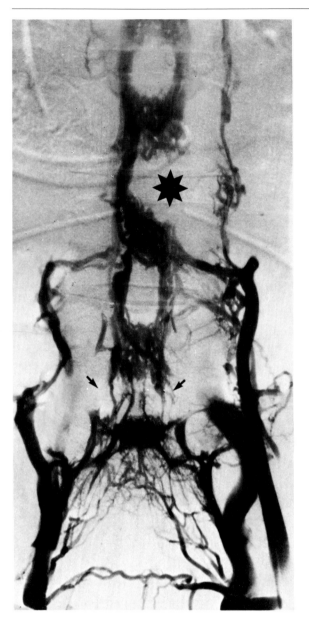

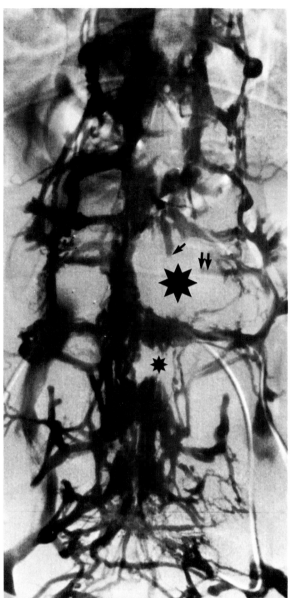

Figure 48

Disc herniation L3–L4 *(star)*. The same phlebogram demonstrates the pathologic pattern of the epidural veins in front of L5–S1 *(arrows)* that corresponded on surgery to another disc herniation. The epidural veins in front of the intermediate disc level L4–L5 are normal

Figure 49

Left disc herniations L4–L5 and L5–S1 *(star)*. In front of L4–L5 the left epidural veins are interrupted *(arrow)* with interruption of the inferior vein of the lateral foramen *(double arrow)*. The clinical symptomatology suggested left L5 sciatica. Nevertheless the same phlebogram showed an interruption of the left epidural veins in front of L5–S1. The excision of the two pathologic discs was performed in the same operation

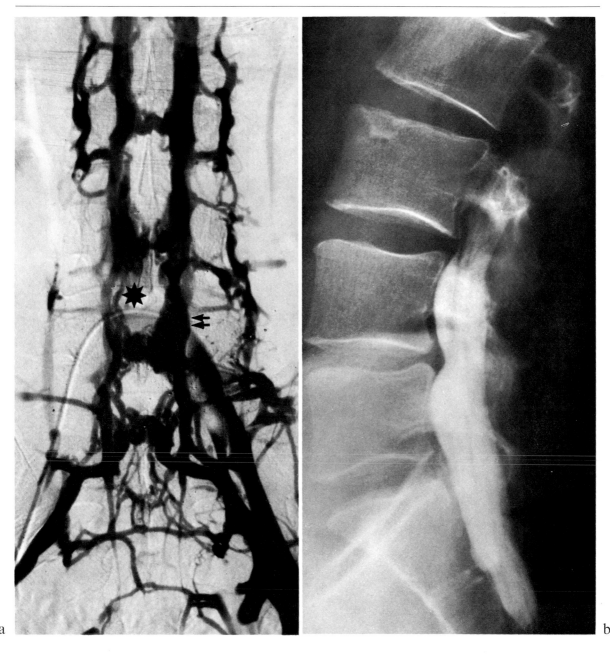

a

b

Figure 50a and b

Midline disc herniation L4–L5

a Phlebogram: asymmetrical wideness of the epidural veins in front of L4–L5 due to slight compression of the right medial epidural vein by the disc lesion situated on the midline *(star)* and to the bypass of the disc obstacle by the venous flow *(double arrow)*

b Radiculogram (Dimer X). Lateral projection. Disc herniation visualized in front of L4–L5

2.4. Lumbar Neuralgia

J. Théron and A. Chevrot

Lumbar neuralgia is a very frequent condition but only a few cases are sufficiently severe and incapacitating to justify radiologic investigations other than routine plain films of the spine.

Clinical examination and plain films of the spine usually quickly indicate a tumoral syndrome or an inflammatory condition of the vertebral body; the radiologic work-up is then different and will not be discussed here. In most cases the radiologist encounters a low back pain syndrome associated or not with a narrow intervertebral space or spaces and with spondylotic formations that are so commonly observed on asymptomatic patients that they can rarely be held responsible for the present symptomatology with any degree of certainty.

If complementary investigations are decided upon, they will be orientated towards the investigation of two main mechanisms that are often connected: a disc lesion and a lesion of the articular facets. In the investigation of a disc lesion, phlebography is a valuable technique, as it is harmless and accurate; but it does not preclude the other techniques of investigation such as radiculography, discography, and diagnostic infiltration of the articular facets.

The clinical history of lumbar neuralgia presents episodes that reflect the various steps of disc degeneration. Acute lumbar neuralgia is due to the clamping of a fragment of nucleus into a tear in the annulus that would be peripheral enough to compress the posterior longitudinal ligament innervated by sensory fibers of the sinu-vertebral nerve (Fig. 51). Chronic lumbar neuralgia would correspond to a similar mechanism but without the clamping of a fragment of the nucleus, presumably because of a wider tear in the annulus. Finally, lumbosciatic neuralgia is due to the issue of disc material through the posterior longitudinal ligament, generally in its weaker lateral portion, with compression of the corresponding nerve root.

In cases of true disc herniation, the clinical expression of which is sciatica or sometimes pure lumbar neuralgia, phlebography, as described in Section 2.3, shows an interruption of the epidural veins in front of the lesion (Fig. 52). In this case, phlebography performed alone or after radiculography will usually provide enough information to orientate the disc excision at the right level. Conversely, when lumbar neuralgia is due to a simple bulging of a fragment of nucleus into a tear in the annulus there is no "true" disc herniation but only chronic or sometimes intermittent irritation of the posterior longitudinal ligament. This kind of lesion does not show up on the phlebogram as dramatically as a true disc herniation. Phlebography frequently provides signs that are indicative but not conclusive; in our experience these signs are morphologic and dynamic.

Morphologic signs are a tortuous and irregular pattern of the epidural veins observed, mainly on the medial ones, in front of the pathologic intervertebral disc with mild localized interruptions, associated or not with dilatation of the venous retrocorporeal anastomosis situated above or below the disc lesion (Figs. 53, 54, 55). These signs are demonstrated on routine phlebograms with compression of the inferior vena cava but may be replaced by a complete interruption of the epidural veins on the series performed without compression that sometimes makes more obvious the effect of a minor bulge on the veins (Fig. 55).

Surgery performed on the basis of these results will sometimes reveal a bulging of the disc but also in some cases a flat but soft and degenerated disc, the excision of which nevertheless gives satisfactory clinical results (see Sect. 2.5). When the results of phlebography are considered insufficiently conclusive, complementary investigations are necessary before performing surgery. Discography is, in our opinion, the best technique provided that the reproduction of the pain is investigated by injection into the nucleus (see technique using neuroleptanalgesia, Sect. 2.9). This test is necessary because, when discography is performed under general anesthesia, it is hardly possible to hold a degenerated disc responsible for the present symptomatology, since such discs are commonly observed even in asymptomatic patients. Discography is also necessary to check the degree of degenerescence of the new disc of junction when intersomatic arthrodesis is decided upon.

While the discal mechanism is the prime factor in the etiology of lumbar neuralgia, the role of lesions of the articular facets should not be forgotten. At the beginning of this century, this lesion was considered chiefly responsible for lumbar neuralgia but was later almost completely abandoned in favor of a discal pathogeny. The pain determined by the articular facets is due to the dorsal ramus of the nerve root (Fig. 51). Modifications of the edges of an articular facet, as observed on an oblique plain film, still do not rule out a secondary or associated lesion of the corresponding disc, and this articular facet cannot with certainty be held responsible for the present symptoms (Fig. 56).

After MASLOW and ROTHMAN [61] in the United States and GINESTIE [45] in France, our radiologic work-up of lumbar neuralgia often now begins with a diagnostic infiltration of the articular facets with xylocaine and steroids. This test should be performed on at least two vertebral levels because of the connection of the nerve fibers of the dorsal ramus between adjacent levels; when positive, the pain presented by the patient disappears in the minutes following infiltration. In this case, radiologic investigations will be discontinued and specific treatment for the articular facets will then be discussed. When the pain persists or is only diminished, a disc lesion will be sought, as seen above (Fig. 56).

Lumbar neuralgia due to spondylolisthesis (see Sect. 2.8) or to lumbar stenosis (see Sect. 2.11) will be discussed in the corresponding chapters, but the radiologic work-up of these conditions also schematically consists in the determination of the extent of epidural compression and in the investigation of an anterior (disc) or a posterior (articular facet) lesion, which could be selectively treated.

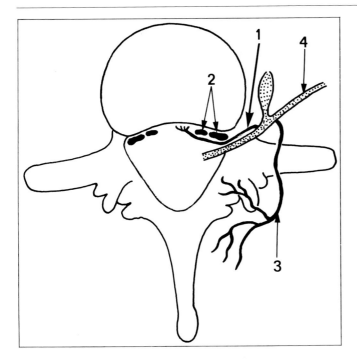

Figure 51

Schematic drawing of the sinuvertebral nerve of Luschka that gives off sensory fibers to the posterior longitudinal ligament, the epidural veins, the dura mater, the bone, and the outer layers of the annulus fibrosus. Note the position of the dorsal ramus of the nerve root that provides sensory fibers to the articular facet

1 Sinuvertebral nerve
2 Epidural veins
3 Dorsal ramus
4 Nerve root
(See also Fig. 18 for the anatomic relationship of the epidural veins to the posterior longitudinal ligament)

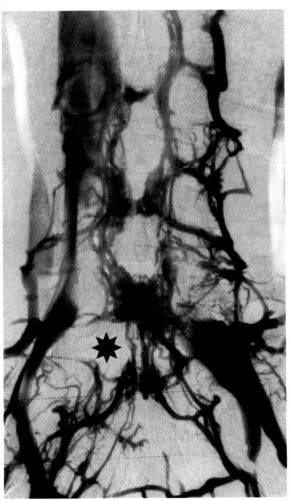

Figure 52

Lumbar neuralgia prevailing on the right side without sciatic irradiation. Phlebogram: interruption of the right lateral epidural vein in front of L5–S1 *(star)*. At surgery: right disc herniation L5–S1

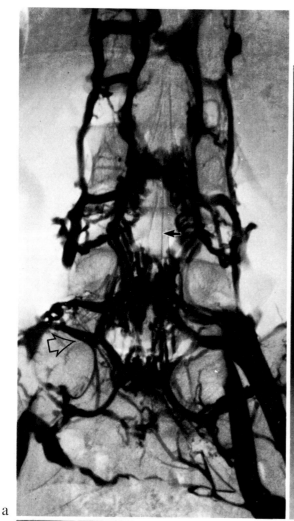

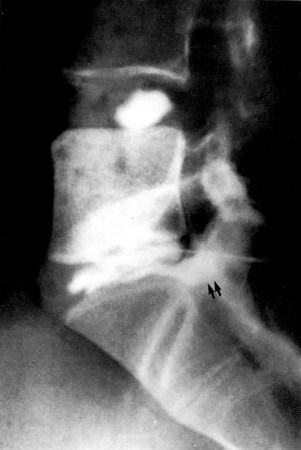

Figure 53a–c

Lumbar neuralgia with transitory irradiation to the left buttock

a Phlebogram: In front of L5–S1 *(large arrow)*, the medial epidural veins appear irregular and tortuous but no obvious interruption is observed. The venous anastomoses below and above this intervertebral disc are mildly dilated. Retrograde filling of a radicular vein is observed, its pathologic significance is still not clear *(arrow)*

b Radiculogram (Dimer X). There is no significant modification of the dural sac and the nerve roots. More particularly the S1 nerve root appears normal *(arrow)*

c Discogram. Injection of the L5–S1 intervertebral disc shows a degenerated nucleus with posterior leakage of the contrast medium *(arrows)*. Conversely, the disc L4–L5 is normal. At surgery: very soft and degenerated intervertebral disc L5–S1; disc excision led to the relief of the lumbar neuralgia

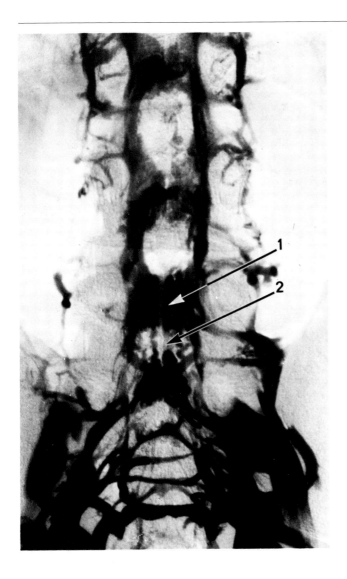

Figure 54

Lumbar neuralgia without sciatic irradiation. Phlebography shows morphologic anomalies in front of L5–S1

1 Venous retrocorporeal anastomoses in front of L5 are markedly dilated
2 Irregular pattern of the medial epidural veins; a short interruption appears in the left one

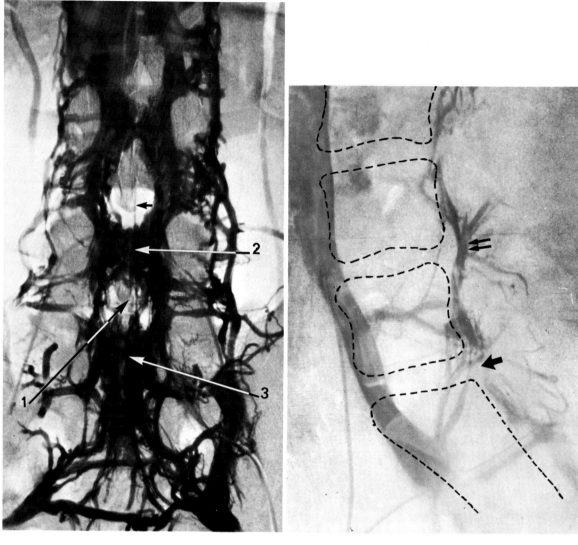

a
b

Figure 55a and b

Lumbar neuralgia without sciatic irradiation

a Phlebogram. AP projection with the routine compression of the inferior vena cava

   1 Mild deformation of the medial epidural veins in front of L5–S1, no venous interruption is observed

   2 Enhancement of the venous retrocorporeal anastomoses in front of L5

   3 Enhancement of the anatomoses in front of S1. Note also the retrograde filling of a radicular vein *(arrow)*; the pathologic significance of this is still not clear

b Same procedure. Lateral projection without compression of the inferior vena cava. An interruption of the epidural veins is observed in front of L5–S1 *(arrow)*. This interruption was not demonstrated on the previous series with compression of the inferior vena cava. Note also the regular posterior displacement of the epidural veins in front of the superior disc L4–L5 *(double arrow)* with no modification of caliber of the veins. This could perhaps illustrate the difference between "nonpathological protrusion" and "disc herniation" (see also Fig. 45)

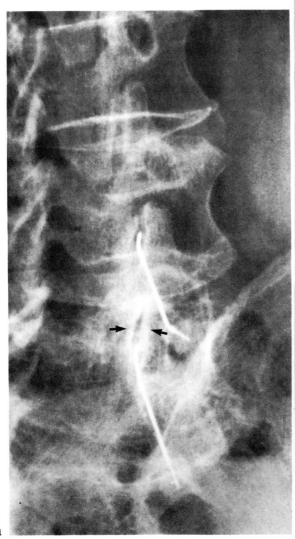

a

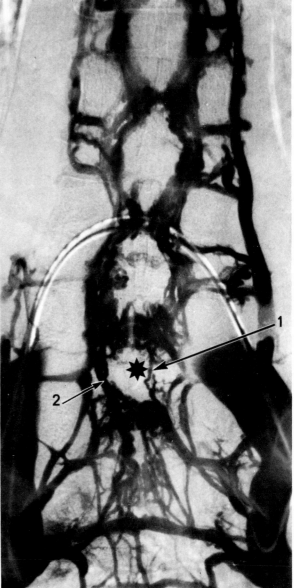

b

Figure 56a and b

Lumbar neuralgia prevailing on the left side without sciatic irradiation. The radiologic exploration included two procedures: infiltration of the left articular facets and lumbar phlebography

a Infiltration of the articular facets L4–L5 and L5–S1. Injection of a steroid and xylocaine into the articular facets did not modify the clinical symptomatology in spite of the bony hyperdensity of the edges of the L5–S1 articular facets *(arrows),* which could have suggested that this articulation was responsible for the lumbar neuralgia

b Phlebogram. Pathologic pattern of the left epidural veins in front of L5–S1
  1 The left medial epidural vein is tortuous and partially interrupted
  2 Slight displacement towards the right side and dilatation of the right medial epidural vein

At surgery: degenerated intervertebral disc L5–S1; disc excision led to the relief of the lumbar neuralgia

2.5. Correlations Between Phlebography and Surgery

J. P. Houtteville

Disc herniations have various clinical presentations that are related not only to their anatomic type but also to individual factors. While there is a common simple type of syndrome with radicular neuralgia due to a disc lesion that is easily recognized and localized, in which case the decision to operate is easily made, there are other types of syndromes where the clinical diagnosis is not so simple. To decide to operate when this is not indicated, or not to operate when it is indicated, are equally serious mistakes.

The usual neuroradiologic techniques do not, in our opinion, provide sufficiently reliable information to help solve this problem, in which the patient's subjective descriptions often constitute a major factor. We have studied a group of 100 patients with disc lesion whom we have personally operated upon, and who have undergone lumbar phlebography performed and interpreted by the same angiographer (Dr. J. THERON); the correlations between phlebography and surgery are presented. They show that phlebography seems to provide very reliable information in the work-up of a disc lesion.

2.5.1. Results of Lumbar Phlebography as Compared to Other Techniques

2.5.1.1. Results of Radiculography (Dimer X)

This technique, classically used before surgery, was performed on 54 patients. In 19 cases, it led to an unequivocal diagnosis of disc herniation. In 12 cases it showed minor signs of radicular compression "not convincing" enough for surgery to be decided upon on their basis alone. In 6 cases it was considered uninterpretable: for anatomic reasons in 3 cases [arachnoid cysts of the nerve sheaths; megadural sac (see Sect. 2.6)] for technical reasons in 2 cases (insufficient filling of the dural sac by contrast medium), and because of postoperative arachnoiditis (see Sect. 2.7) in one case.

In this series radiculography did not provide enough information in 42% of the cases. It allowed the unequivocal diagnosis of disc herniation in 35% of the cases; but this becomes 57% if the 12% of "not convincing" (in our opinion) radiculograms are added.

2.5.1.2. Results of Discography

Only five patients have undergone discography. In each case it showed a posterior leakage of the contrast medium and degeneration of the disc in front of which the veins were interrupted on the phlebogram. The test of reproduction of the pain by injection into the disc was not carried out in this series because the procedures were performed under general anesthesia. The technique of discography has recently been modified with use of neuroleptanalgesia that permits the investigation of reproduction of the pain and consequently provides more information (for technique, see Sect. 2.9).

2.5.1.3. Results of Phlebography

The disc herniation was demonstrated by phlebography in 99 of the cases in the series. In the remaining case, the diagnosis could not be made because the epidural veins could not be injected due to anomalies of the extravertebral veins. Thus, phlebography appears to be the most reliable technique for the work-up of a disc herniation; it is much more reliable than radiculography and gives as much information as discography while having the advantage of being an indirect, harmless, and almost painless technique.

2.5.2. New Information Provided by Phlebography

2.5.2.1. Bilaterality of the Disc Herniation

At the time of intervention, 8 patients had, or had previously had, bilateral sciatica. In every case, phlebography showed bilateral interruption of the veins in front of the pathologic disc. In 11 patients who had only unilateral sciatica, phlebography showed bilateral interruption of the veins.

Surgical correlations: In these 19 cases a bilateral disc herniation was demonstrated at surgery before disc excision. The disc herniation was always more prominent on the painful side when sciatica was unilateral. From a technical point of view this kind of phlebographic information should in our opinion indicate a bilateral surgical approach to the pathologic disc and complete bilateral excision, removing degenerated disc material that could otherwise cause a recurrence of the herniation.

2.5.2.2. Multiple Pathologic Discs

In 23 out of 24 patients, phlebography showed interruption of the epidural veins in front of two discs, and of three discs in the remaining case. This phlebographic information obtained on patients who presented with sciatica, cruralgia, or even pure lumbar neuralgia (4 cases) led us to investigate surgically the discs that appeared pathologic. In 6 patients, we

considered that the intraoperative pattern of one of these discs was normal and left it in place. Of these patients, 5 have not presented any persisting painful syndrome in a follow-up ranging from 6 months to 2 years; however, a further operation was performed on 1 patient 6 months later to excise a disc indicated by phlebography but left in place at the first operation.

In the 16 other cases disc excision was performed at the level indicated by phlebography because intraoperative inspection showed a disc protrusion and/or an abnormal softness when pressed with an instrument. In no case did a thorough follow-up show any painful residual syndrome.

Finally, in two cases we did not think it surgically necessary to examine a disc indicated by phlebography. In the first case, the patient presented with crural neuralgia, and phlebography showed an interruption of the veins in front of L4–L5 by a herniation that compressed the L4 nerve root as demonstrated at surgery; but phlebography also showed an interruption of the veins in front of L5–S1, and nothing in the symptomatology indicated this disc level. The second case was a left disc herniation L4–L5 demonstrated on the phlebogram that also showed a venous interruption in front of L5–S1 on the right side, which had never been painful.

This 24% of cases in which phlebography showed multiple apparently pathologic discs deserves more thorough reflection: Are they false positive errors, as could suggest the six cases in which surgical inspection showed no significant change of the disc? However, we saw that in one of these cases a further operation was necessary for excision of a disc left in place at the first operation. Is it, on the other hand, a major indication when phlebography shows several pathologic discs in a patient who apparently presents at only one level with a painful disc syndrome? Is the excision of the discs indicated by phlebography the best method of prevention of residual lumbar neuralgia? Our series is too small to confirm this hypothesis but the question remains open as long as, the overall results of the surgical treatment of disc lesions show a 20% incidence of residual lumbar neuralgia.

2.5.2.3. "Soft Disc"

There are cases in which the clinical history and physical examination indicate a disc herniation but radiculography is negative and phlebography shows a venous interruption in front of a disc that may or may not be clinically suspect. The surgeon finds a disc which is not bulging but which, when palpated with an instrument, feels soft. When the posterior longitudinal ligament is cut, the disc substance, markedly degenerated and almost liquid, comes out under pressure and disc excision leads to the relief of the painful syndrome.

We had eight of cases of this nature. Here again, phlebography provided important information for making the decision to operate (successfully in each case) on patients whom radiculography (negative in each case) would have led us to consider "functional", and who did not have a "true" disc herniation but nevertheless suffered from algogenic discopathy that presumably was expressed only on certain strains or movements.

2.5.2.4. Lumbar Neuralgia

The pathogeny of lumbar neuralgia is difficult to establish with precision: Is it determined by a disc lesion or by the articular facets? Should it be treated by disc excision when a disc lesion is apparent? Which surgical technique should be used: disc excision or intersomatic arthrodesis from an anterior approach? It is not our purpose to answer all these questions but the major problem, in our opinion, remains to ascertain a discopathy; and here again phlebography seems to be very helpful.

Out of 12 cases, the clinical symptomatology was pure lumbar neuralgia in 4 and lumbar neuralgia with intermittent or hardly localized sciatic irradiation in the remainder. On phlebography, the venous interruption was shown to be bilateral in 7 cases and unilateral in 5. In 2 cases two discs were demonstrated as pathologic on phlebography. Surgery oriented by phlebography consisted in the excision of the indicated discs; up to the time of writing, no patient has presented with any residual painful syndrome.

2.5.3. Advantages of Phlebography

The technical conditions for performing phlebography have been very useful on several occasions:

2.5.3.1. Emergency Surgery

It is possible to operate on patients in the genupectoral position immediately after phlebography. This cannot be done after radiculography with dimer X, since it is necessary to wait a little for resorption of the contrast. This was useful in three cases of sciatics with palsy; we could operate within 6 h following the beginning of the deficit and consequently there was a better chance of neural recuperation.

2.5.3.2. Hyperalgic Sciatica

Phlebography is performed on the patient in the supine position and is thus better tolerated than radiculography, which necessitates the upright position (two cases); for the same reason phlebography was preferred to radiculography for a patient who vanished when lumbar puncture was attempted.

2.5.3.3. Patients Who Have Previously Undergone Radiculography

Injection of dimer X can provoke arachnoiditis (possibly worsened by disc excision), which prevents accurate interpretation of radiculography. Phlebography will then provide important information (see Sect. 2.7) (one case).

2.5.4. Intraoperative Pattern of the Epidural Veins

We have tried to compare the phlebographic and intraoperative pattern of the epidural veins by using the optic magnification of the surgical microscope. The epidural veins appear variously depending on the patient and on the degree of venous repletion, but their relationships with the disc herniation can be clearly demonstrated. In some cases, the compressed epidural veins "disappear" at the inferior and superior boundaries of the pathologic disc; less frequently their lumen appears flattened by the herniation (Fig. 57).

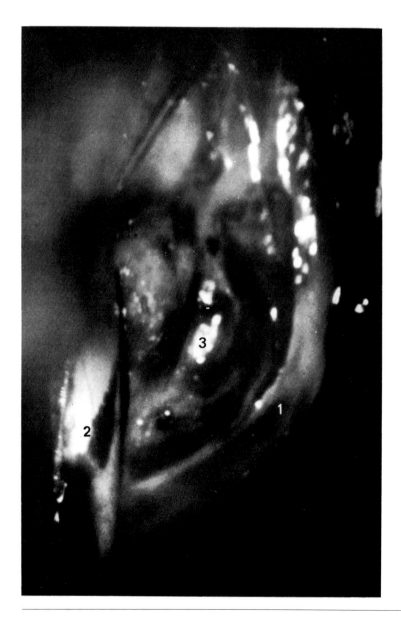

Figure 57

Microsurgical view of a disc herniation compressing the corresponding nerve root and epidural vein

1 Epidural vein flattened by the disc herniation
2 Nerve root
3 Disc herniation

2.6. Megadural Lumbar Sac

L. Picard, J. Roland and D. Larde

The diagnosis of lumbar disc lesions is particularly difficult to make in cases of megadural sac. In our opinion, lumbar phlebography represents a major improvement in facilitating their accurate location.

2.6.1. Radiologic Diagnosis

Plain films give a first indication by showing enlarged dimensions of the lumbar canal but in fact the classic conception of megadural sac should be replaced by the conception of "relatively large" dural sac when its frontal and sagittal diameters are considered. KOMMINOTH and WORINGER [53] described a measurement that compares the interpedicular distance and the dimension of the dural sac in front of L5 on a myelogram. The ratio is normally bigger than 1.5 and goes down close

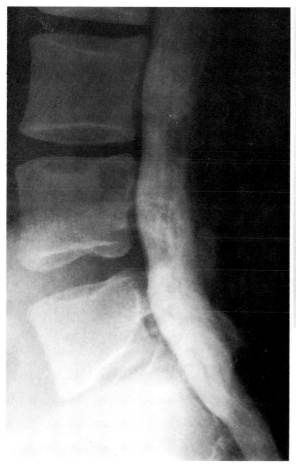

a

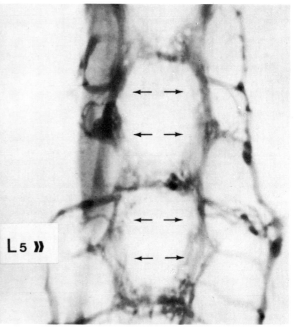

b

Figure 58

a Megadural sac as observed on a lateral radiculogram
b Increased distance between the epidural veins *(arrows)* presenting a characteristic rectangular pattern

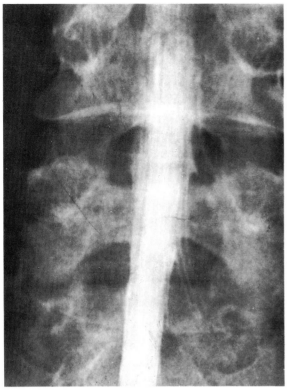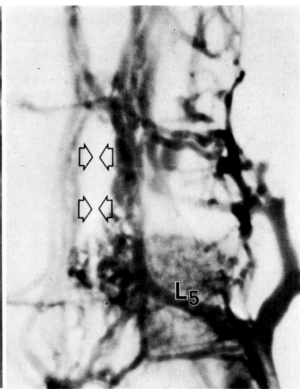

a   b

Figure 59

a "Narrow" dural sac as observed on an AP radiculogram
b Shortening of the distance between the epidural veins
  (arrows)

to 1 in the case of megadural sac. Lumbar phlebography is an indirect technique, but it nevertheless provides quite characteristic results: The distance between the longitudinal epidural veins of each side appears increased and the veins are more linear and stretched, together forming a rectangle (Fig. 58). These modifications should be compared to the fusiform pattern of the epidural veins observed in stenosis of the lumbar canal (Fig. 59) (see also Sect. 2.11).

2.6.2. Lumbar Disc Lesions and Megadural Sac

In our own series of 18 patients presenting megadural sac revealed by radiculography,

which was performed as the first technique of investigation, phlebography demonstrated in 8 patients a disc lesion that was not seen on the radiculogram (Fig. 60).

The false negative cases in radiculography have often been erroneously attributed to the use of an insufficient amount of contrast medium; this can be avoided by the use of better tolerated contrast medium such as Amipaque, but overfilling of the dural sac can also be misleading in concealing the lesions behind too dense an opacity.

In cases of megadural sac, lumbar phlebography demonstrates most clearly its superiority to radiculography for the diagnosis of disc lesions.

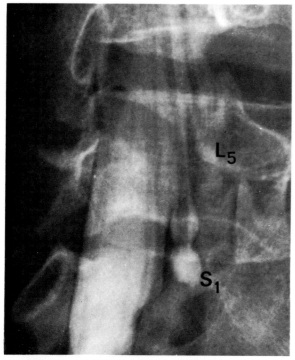

a

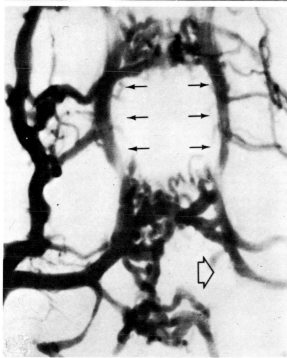

b

Figure 60a and b

Left sciatica S1

a Radiculogram, oblique projection. Megadural sac with radicular cysts

b Phlebogram. Increased distance between the epidural veins due to the megadural sac *(arrows)*. Interruption of the left epidural veins in front of L5–S1 *(open arrow)* due to disc herniation

2.7. Arachnoiditis, Epiduritis

L. Picard, J. Roland, D. Larde and P. Blanchot

The lesions of arachnoiditis of the dural sac as observed on a radiculogram are now better known; they vary in origin (infiltration, radiculography, myelography, infectious disease, surgery). They can involve the various spaces or meninges, giving rise to the distinction between arachnoiditis, epiduritis, and arachnoepiduritis, which are similar as regards clinical presentation. Phlebography provides complementary and sometimes better information than does radiculography in their investigation.

2.7.1. Arachnoiditis

Isolated inflammatory lesions of the arachnoid membrane do not modify the epidural veins; the phlebogram in pure arachnoiditis is normal in spite of the major modifications observed on the radiculogram (Fig. 61). It is in pure arachnoiditis that phlebography provides better information than radiculography, which shows marked modifications that preclude the accurate diagnosis of a recurrent disc lesion.

2.7.2. Epiduritis

Inflammation of the epidural space always determines localized modifications of the veins which appear irregular and often interrupted; the phlebogram shows venous modifications quite identical to those observed in arachnoepiduritis but on the radiculogram the nerve roots appear normal in a dural sac narrowed by epiduritis. When epiduritis occurs after surgery, the interruption of the epidural veins due to the operation makes the diagnosis of recurrent disc herniation even more difficult.

2.7.3. Arachnoepiduritis

These major lesions form extensive inflammatory scars, the radiologic signs of which combine the signs of arachnoiditis on radiculography and of epiduritis on phlebography. In most cases they follow surgery and are more frequently observed after laminectomy. It is almost impossible to make the diagnosis of recurrence of a disc herniation from a phlebogram because of the severity of the venous modifications (Figs. 62 and 63).

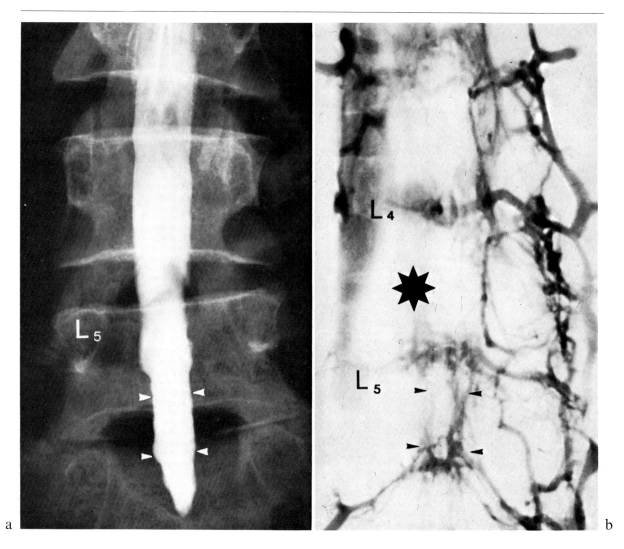

a

b

Figure 61

a Second radiculogram (dimer X). Patient's history includes infiltrations. Severe arachnoiditis with rigidity, hyperdensity, and narrowing of the dural sac below L3. Nerve root emergences are not distinguishable

b Phlebogram. Poor opacification of epidural veins due to unilateral injection. Subnormal pattern of L5–S1 epidural veins *(arrowheads)*. Interruption of the right epidural veins in front of L4–L5 due to disc herniation *(star)*. Phlebography has in this case provided more information than radiculography

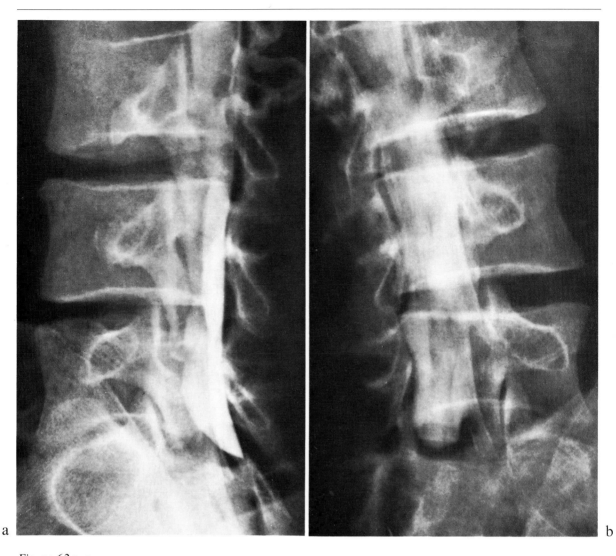

a

b

Figure 62a–c

Surgery for right disc herniation L4–L5 3 months previously

a Radiculogram. Right posterior oblique projection. Marked arachnoepiduritis. Nerve roots are not distinguishable on this side

b Same procedure. Left posterior oblique projection. Dural sac is shortened but the nerve roots are observed on this side

c Phlebogram. Normal pattern of epidural veins on the left side. No opacification of the veins in front of L4–L5; poor filling in front of L5–S1

At surgery: marked arachnoepiduritis on right side

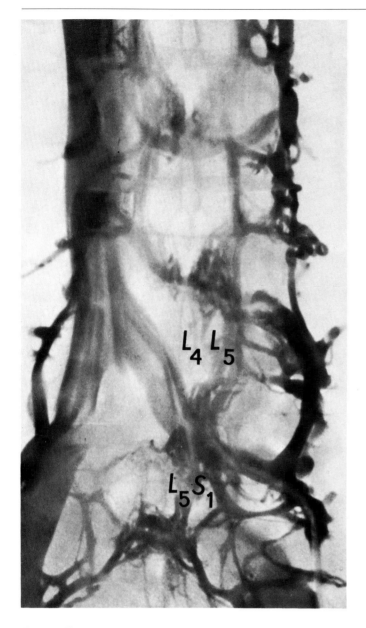

Figure 62c (legend see p. 77)

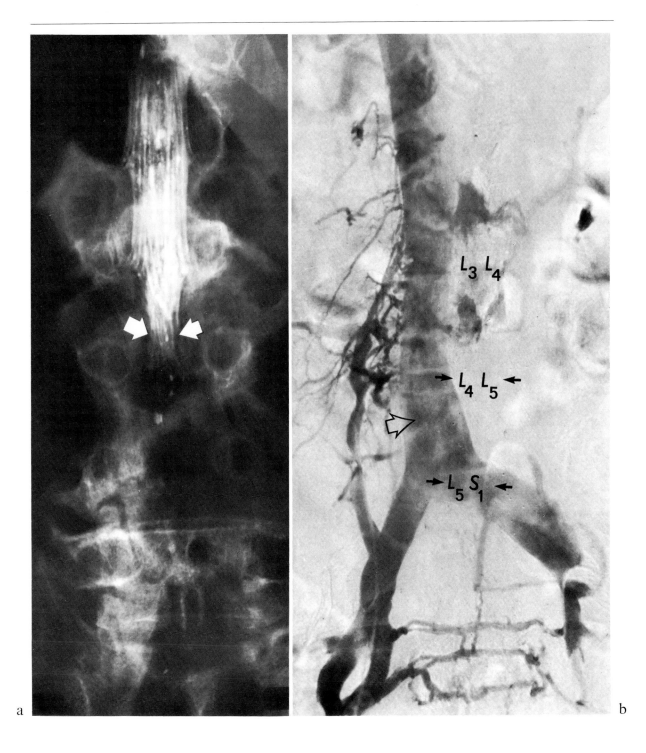

a   b

Figure 63a and b

Previous surgery for L4–L5 disc herniation

a Radiculogram. The dural sac cannot be opacified below
   L3 *(arrows)*

b Phlebogram. Epidural veins cannot be opacified in front
   of L4–L5 and L5–S1 *(arrows)* due to marked postoperative arachnoepiduritis. Note the reflux in the inferior
   vena cava *(open arrow)*.

2.8. Spondylolisthesis

J. Moret and H. Ammerich

Spondylolisthesis is an anterior sliding of a vertebral body on the underlying vertebra; it is a fairly common condition, affecting 2%–3% of the population. Leaving aside here post-traumatic spondylolisthesis due to isthmic fracture, two types of spondylolisthesis can be described:

— True spondylolisthesis with congenital isthmic defect [35]
— Pseudospondylolisthesis with intact posterior arch [18, 36, 73]

Spondylolisthesis involves the lumbosacral junction in 80% of cases and in 11% the L4–L5 intervertebral space. In rare cases it involves the L3–L4 or L2–L3 interspace, and may involve two intervertebral spaces.

A patient with spondylolisthesis usually presents clinically with bilateral or unilaterally predominant lumbosacralgia; lumbosciatic neuralgia, which may involve one side or the other intermittently is also found. There is no correlation between the intensity of the clinical signs and the anatomic severity of the spondylolisthesis. Our purpose is to compare the information provided by phlebography and by other radiologic techniques usually performed in the work-up of spondylolisthesis [62].

From a technical point of view, phlebography is performed in most cases as usual (see Sect. 2.2) but it is frequently necessary to perform two different series with catheterization of an ascending lumbar vein and of a lateral sacral vein for the first series, and of two lateral sacral veins for the second; this usually provides better information on the epi-dural veins situated in front of L5–S1, which are most frequently involved, and on the veins of the lateral foramen at the level of spondylolisthesis and of the levels above and below.

It can also be useful to perform "dynamic" series with injection in the upright position or after correction of hyperlordosis with a pillow; injection is then performed, keeping the same compression of the vena cava, and the same amount and rate of contrast medium as used in the routine series. This dynamic series can show modifications in venous filling as compared to the phlebogram in standard dorsal decubitus position; these modifications should be considered pathologic and related to vertebral sliding, since in normal patients there is no modification of venous filling between the upright and decubitus positions (the series are performed under nonphysiologic conditions).

2.8.1. Phlebographic Results

These results are usually related to the stretching of the epidural veins on the posterior edge of the superior plate of the underlying vertebra (usually S1); an interruption of the veins is then observed on the phlebogram. The epidural veins can also be interrupted by posterior compression applied by the fibrous sleeve around the isthmic defect and by hypertrophy of the articular facets and laminas with thickening of the ligamenta flava. These various lesions consequently form an AP stenosis of the spinal canal which predominates in the lateral recessus and lateral foramen. This narrowing is responsible for the ischemic claudication of the pseudovascular syndrome, which is observed mainly in pseudospondylolisthesis with intact posterior arch.

The location of the epidural veins in contact with the vertebral body and attached to the posterior longitudinal vertebral ligament explains the good correlation of the phlebographic signs and the severity of vertebral sliding. The following classification can be proposed:

Stage I. No interruption of the epidural veins (Figs. 64a and 65). It is however possible to localize the level of spondylolisthesis because of the marked shortening of the distance between the venous anastomoses. This shortening (due to the sliding of the superior vertebra) should be appreciated relative to the normal shortening of the veins in front of L5–S1 on AP routine phlebograms due to the normal sacral posterior tilting.

Stage II. Bilateral and symmetrical interruption of the lateral epidural veins, sometimes with displacement of the medial ones (Figs. 64b, 66a, b, c).

Stage III. Bilateral and symmetrical interruption of the lateral and medial epidural veins (Figs. 64c, 67).

At each of these different stages a complete or partial interruption of the veins of the lateral foramen can be observed, directly related to the modifications of the posterior arch, as seen above, that narrow and compress the inside of the lateral recess and lateral foramen (Fig. 66a and c). To these phlebographic signs, directly related to spondylolisthesis, can be also added the modifications of the epidural veins determined by an associated disc herniation usually arising on the superior intervertebral disc because at the level of spondylolisthesis a disc herniation is quite rare (Figs. 64e, 68).

The diagnosis of spondylolisthesis is made from the plain films but phlebography provides major information on the exact site and extent of compression of the epidural space and nerve roots due to vertebral sliding and also shows associated disc herniations. In permitting a better understanding of the lesions it facilitates treatment.

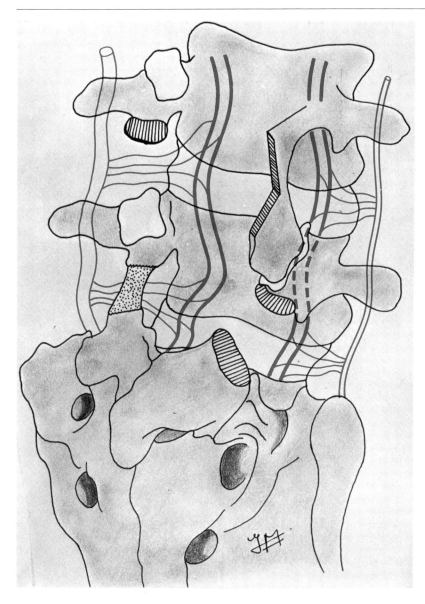

Figure 64a

Spondylolisthesis, stage 1. Normal pattern of epidural veins

Figure 64a–d

The various phlebographic signs encountered in spondylolisthesis, represented on a posterior right oblique projection of the lumbosacral area
Dotted area, isthmic dehiscence area. *hatched area,* section of posterior columns (for ledgibility). *Black dots,* interruption of the veins of the lateral foramina that can be seen in any type of spondylolisthesis

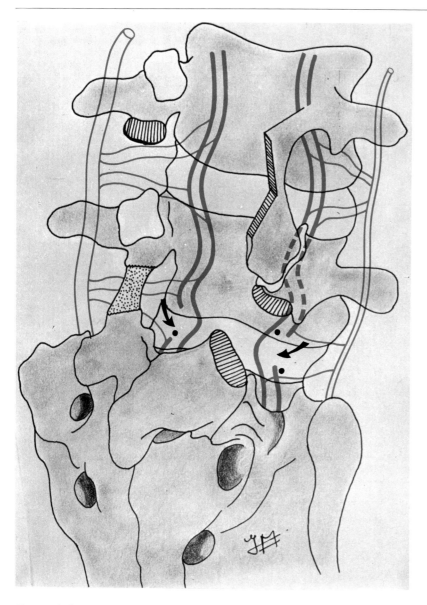

Figure 64b

Spondylolisthesis, stage 2. Bilateral and symmetrical interruption of lateral epidural veins *(curved arrows)* usually associated with medial displacement of the medial epidural veins

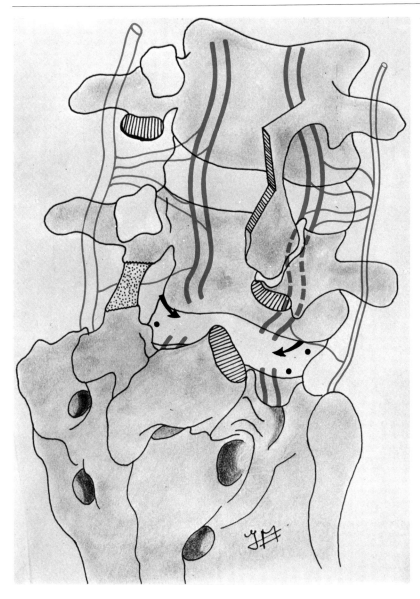

Figure 64c

Spondylolisthesis, stage 3. Bilateral interruption of epidural veins

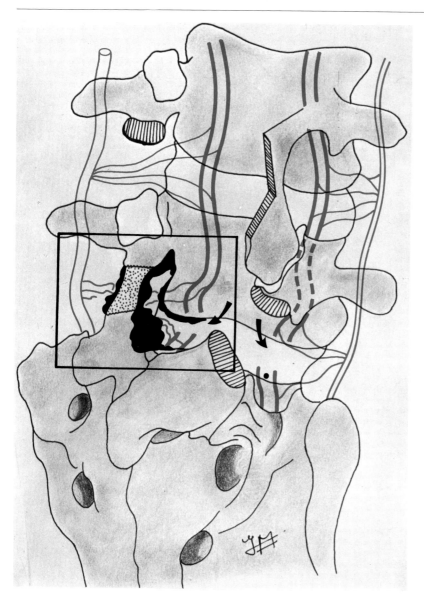

Figure 64 d

Schematic drawing (inset) of secondary degenerative modifications *(black)* of the posterior column and vertebral body that narrow the lateral recessus of the spinal canal and the corresponding lateral foramen

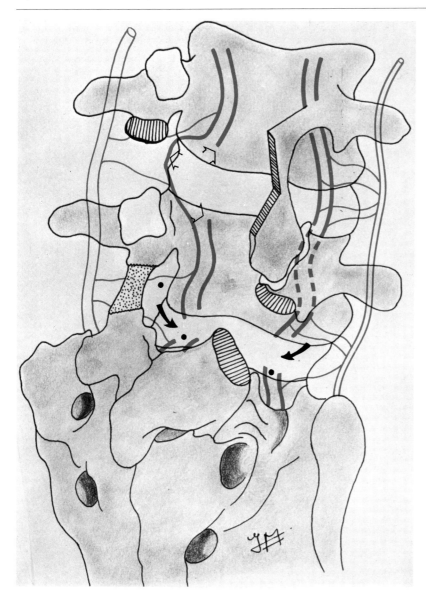

Figure 64e

Association of L5–S1 spondylolisthesis, stage 3 *(curved arrows)* with a left L4–L5 disc herniation that interrupts the medial epidural vein and displaces laterally the lateral epidural vein *(open arrow)*.

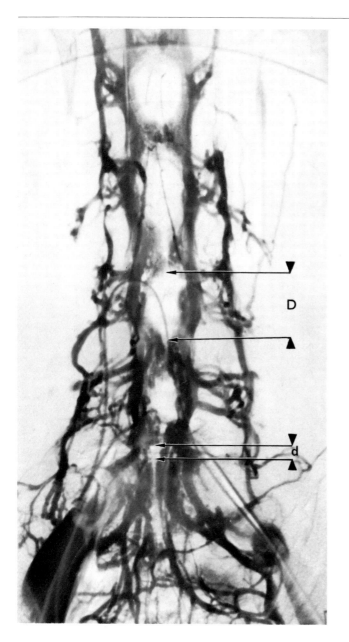

Figure 65

Spondylolisthesis, stage 1. No interruption of epidural veins is observed. However the level of the spondylolisthesis (L5–S1) can be recognized because of the marked shortening of the distance between venous anastomoses *(d/D)*. This shortening (due to vertebral sliding) should be appreciated proportionally to normal shortening of the veins in front of L5–S1 on AP phlebograms due to sacral posterior tilting.

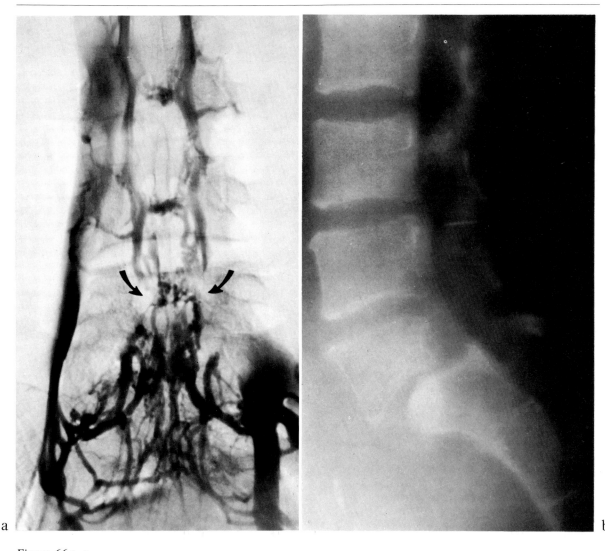

a

b

Figure 66 a–c

a and c. Spinal phlebograms performed on two different
   patients with stage-2 spondylolisthesis. Note characteristic interruption of lateral epidural veins *(curved ar-*
   rows). Phlebograms have been performed via bilateral
   sacral veins catheterization and the non opacification
   of the veins of the lateral foramen is interpreted as
   pathologic only when it persists after complementary
   ascending lumbar vein injection

b Air myelogram of the patient whose phlebogram is represented on (a)

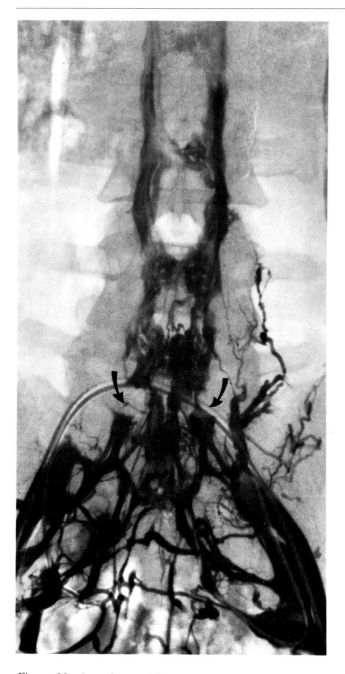

Figure 66 c (legend see p. 89)

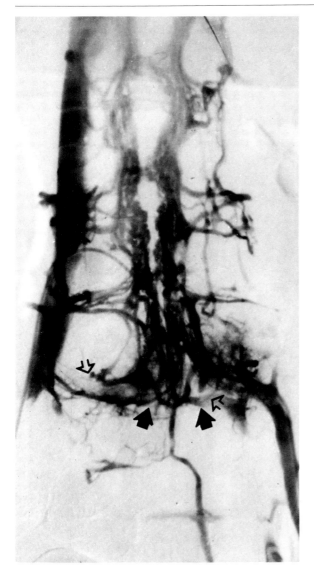

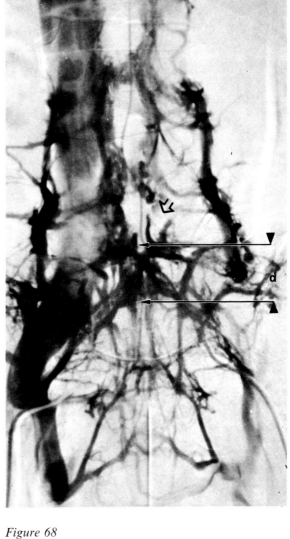

Figure 67

L5–S1 spondylolisthesis, stage 3 with bilateral interruption of epidural veins *(black arrows)*. Association with interruption of the veins of the foramen *(open arrows)*

Figure 68

L5–S1 spondylolisthesis, stage 1. Note the flattening of the characteristic "lozenge" pattern of the phlebogram at this level *(d)*. Association with a left disc herniation at L4–L5 level, interrupting the epidural veins *(open arrow)*

2.9. Phlebography in Conjunction with Discography

J. F. Ginestie

With the collaboration of B. Fassio, C. Buscayret, H. Connes, J.P. Bouvier, and J. Vidal

Lumbar neuralgia and sciatica that does not respond to medical treatment often represents a difficult diagnostic and therapeutic problem. Traumatic, neurologic, tumoral, and infectious etiologies will not be considered here, since they are rare and are differently managed. For the other types of lumbosciatic neuralgia, which are much more frequent, the problem is too often limited to investigation and treatment of any disc lesion; this partially explains the occasional bad surgical results and the rather large number of patients for whom no definitive treatment is proposed.

Many factors, individually or associated with a disc lesion, can be responsible for lumbar neuralgia or lumbosciatic neuralgia; research into the most complete work-up of these "surgical" cases led us to propose the use of phlebography in conjunction with discography which, in our opinion, affords many advantages.

2.9.1. Lumbar Phlebography

2.9.1.1. Advantages

By the visualization of the epidural veins, phlebography allows a good study of the right and left anterolateral portions of the spinal canal. It is an indirect technique that provides major information on disc herniations (see Sect. 2.3), inflammatory lesions of the epidural space (see Sect. 2.7) and stenosis of the lumbar canal (see Sect. 2.11). By opacifying the veins of the lateral foramen, it permits good analysis of any lateral extension of the lesion.

2.9.1.2. Limitations for Disc Pathology

False negative cases are exceptional with phlebography but may occur regarding herniations above L5–S1 (see Sect. 2.3).

Phlebography accurately shows the site of venous compression but gives only approximate information on the degree of degeneration of the other discs (see Sect. 2.4): This information is essential in the work-up of lumbar neuralgia, particularly when arthrodesis is decided upon.

Nonopacification of the veins of a lateral foramen above an interruption of the epidural veins has no diagnostic value.

Venous interruption in front of an intervertebral disc already excised can be related to the coagulation of the epidural veins during surgery and is of no value for the diagnosis of recurrence of a disc herniation at this level.

2.9.2. Discography

2.9.2.1. Advantages

Discography opacifies the nucleus of the pathologic disc and thus provides precise information on its degree of degeneration.

The reproduction of the pain by injection into the pathologic disc allows the determination of the disc responsible for the painful syndrome.

The discs situated above and below the pathologic disc can be examined.

2.9.2.2. Limitations

Discography only provides information on disc pathology.

The contrast medium does not immediately mix with the gelatinous substance of the nucleus but accumulates inside or threads its way between the nucleus, the annulus, and the vertebral plates. This explains the variety in appearance of a normal disc on early films, but the pictures are all similar when late films are taken (after the 12th hour).

In cases of disc herniation, the contrast medium leaks into the epidural space through the weakest portions of the disc; this can be on the side of the herniation, which then presents as lacunas in the contrast medium or on the opposite side, and the herniation cannot be localized on the discogram.

2.9.3. Combined Use of Phlebography and Discography

2.9.3.1. Advantages

As seen above, each of the two techniques provides complementary information where the other is inadequate. This was why we decided to use them conjointly.

In disc pathology a significant interruption of the epidural veins indicates the site of compression but when the veins are only slightly displaced or not significantly interrupted, discography permits this to be ascertained (Fig. 69a, b, c). Discography consequently eliminates the rare false negative cases in phlebography and permits the degree of degeneration of the other discs to be established. Phlebography completes the investigation by showing any extension of disc material into the lateral foramen.

2.9.3.2. Limitations

Only epidural-space pathology is investigated; other frequent etiologies of painful syndromes, such as a facet syndrome (see Sect. 2.4) cannot be shown.

2.9.4. Techniques

Phlebography and discography are performed at the same time; so the patient undergoes only one procedure and the radiologist obtains a maximum of information. The procedure is performed under neuroleptanalgesia and begins with phlebography to avoid the superimposition of the veins and of an injected disc or a long-lasting leakage of contrast medium into the epidural space. Discography is then performed with the patient in the lateral decubitus position. The discs are punctured and then neuroleptanalgesia is reduced to investigate the reproduction of the pain by injection into the pathologic disc.

2.9.5. Indications

2.9.5.1. Lumbar Neuralgia (see also Sect. 2.4)

Use of phlebography and discography in conjunction is indicated when the lumbar neuralgia is chronic or recurrent and resists medical treatment. However, after the routine plain films, we begin by investigating the possibility of an articular facet syndrome by arthrography and diagnostic infiltration of the posterior articulations; this technique is the simplest of the special procedures of investigation of the lumbar spine. When this gives negative or only partially positive results, we prefer a conjunction of phlebography and discography to discography alone for the reasons stated above.

---▷

Figure 69a–c

a Phlebogram. Interruption of the left medial epidural vein *(arrow)* in front of L5–S1 with enlargement of the contralateral right medial vein. These two signs make the diagnosis of L5–S1 disc lesion quite certain. Conversely the epidural veins in front of L4–L5 are not definitely interrupted but the venous strip seems thinner on the right and the venous anastomosis in front of L4 appears slightly dilated. An L4–L5 disc lesion may be suspected on phlebographic evidence, but the diagnosis is not certain

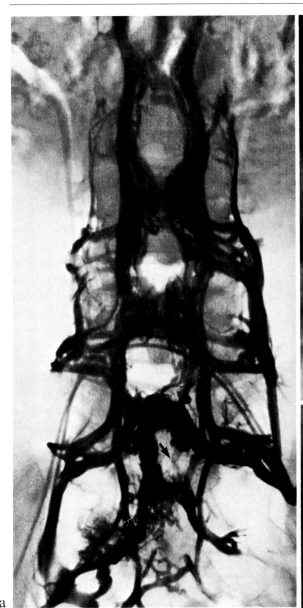

a

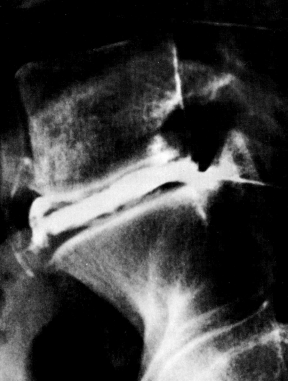

b

Figure 69 a–c

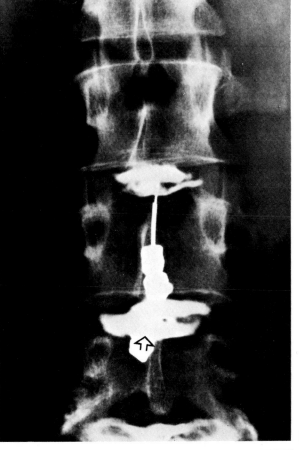

c

b Discogram L5–S1—lateral projection. The disc L5–S1 appears degenerated with leakage of the contrast medium anteriorly and posteriorly. The results of phlebography are thus confirmed

c *Discogram L3–L4, L4–L5, and L5–S1—AP projection. The disc L3–L4 appears normal. The disc L5–S1, as seen on B is markedly degenerated. The disc L4–L5 arrow is not as degenerated as L5–S1 but the nucleus appears larger than normal; this disc presents a certain degree of degeneration that corresponds to the mild modifications of the epidural veins shown on the phlebogram*

2.9.5.2. Lumbosciatic Neuralgia
(see also Sect. 2.3)

The patient presents with sciatica associated with homolateral lumbar neuralgia but many episodes of lumbar neuralgia can usually be found in the history. Joint use of phlebography and discography is, in our opinion, the best method of investigation for the purpose of planning surgery. When this technique is negative, we then inject the articular facets as seen above.

2.9.5.3. Spondylolisthesis (see also Sect. 2.8)

When surgical treatment is decided upon, discography is necessary to visualize the degree of degeneration of the disc at the level of spondylolisthesis and at the level situated above it, which will become the new disc of junction after the operation. Phlebography provides complementary information on the degree of vertebral sliding and on the compression of the inside of the lateral foramen, and this indicates whether a reduction of the displacement is necessary in the cases with minor sliding.

2.9.6. Contraindications

There are no contraindications to discography but we prefer not to use phlebography on patients with a history of thrombophlebitis, to avoid thrombotic complications (see Sect. 2.2).

2.9.7. Conclusion

The use of phlebography and discography in conjunction provides a maximum of information when performed at the same time in the work-up of a painful syndrome of the lumbar spine because their respective diagnostic possibilities are complementary.

2.10. Tumors

J. Théron and J. Moret

For anatomic and technical reasons, lumbar phlebography is of less interest in the field of tumor pathology than in that of disc pathology. In Section 2.1 it was shown that the classic description of two anterior and two posterior longitudinal veins is wrong: The four longitudinal veins are located in the anterolateral angles of the spinal canal and thus represent a good landmark for study of the lesions developed in the anterior side of the canal or large enough to compress the anterior epidural space. Conversely, the epidural veins can remain unaffected by small tumors that develop in the posterior portion of the canal (Fig. 70a and b) or by tumors hanging from the roots of the cauda equina that do not compress the anterior epidural space (Fig. 71).

Technically, phlebography usually takes longer than myelography and needs an experienced angiographer, angiographic equipment, and a trained team of technicians. Furthermore, when a tumor is very large the superior limit of compression is sometimes not shown on the phlebogram, and complementary myelography via suboccipital puncture is then necessary.

Nevertheless, phlebography has some advantages: it does not introduce contrast medium into the subarachnoid spaces and can provide useful information on any extravertebral extension of the tumor (Figs. 72, 73).

The phlebographic signs of a tumor are not specific and a tumoral compression is here again marked by localized or extensive absence of opacification of the epidural veins. When the tumor is large enough to compress the anterior epidural space, the veins are interrupted at the same site as the arrest of the contrast medium on the myelogram (Fig. 74). In the case of a smaller lesion the modification of the veins is different depending on the speed of growth of the lesion: When the tumor grows rapidly, the epidural veins are rapidly compressed and appear interrupted on the phlebogram; conversely, when the tumor grows slowly, particularly if it has been present since infancy, the epidural veins can adapt their shape to the growth of the tumor and mold themselves to it without being interrupted (Fig. 72). Finally the negative results of phlebography in the case of tumors that do not compress the anterior epidural space has already been mentioned above.

In practice, phlebography should not be used as the first contrast technique to study a tumor developed in the spinal canal. When a lumbar tumor is suspected, myelography should be used. We, nevertheless, use phlebography in two circumstances: (1) When spinal-cord angiography is performed under general anesthesia to study the vascularization of the tumor, phlebography is performed at the same time and as seen above, sometimes provides complementary information without subjecting the patient to another procedure. (2) When a retroperitoneal tumor is presumed to extend intravertebrally (Neuroblastoma) in a young child; aortography is here again performed at the same time as phlebography (technically easy in young children) and information on the extra- and intravertebral extension of the lesion are thus obtained. Complementary myelography is not usually necessary and surgery can be performed according to the results of pyelography, aortography, and phlebography (Fig. 75).

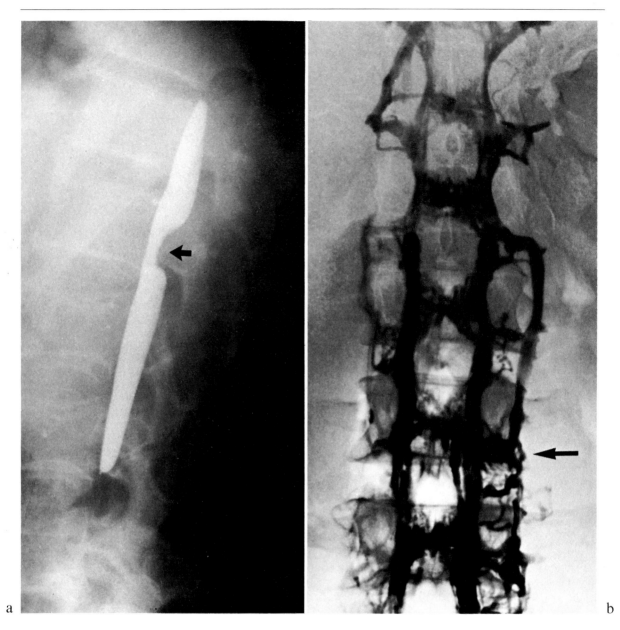

a

b

Figure 70a and b

Lumbar meningioma

a Opaque myelography (Duroliopaque)—lateral projection. A tumor is demonstrated on the posterior side of the spinal canal *(arrow)*

b Lumbar phlebogram. AP projection. Normal pattern of the epidural veins in front of the tumor *(arrow)* due to the anterior position of the epidural veins in the spinal canal. This explains the weakness of phlebography in cases of a tumor situated posteriorly in the spinal canal

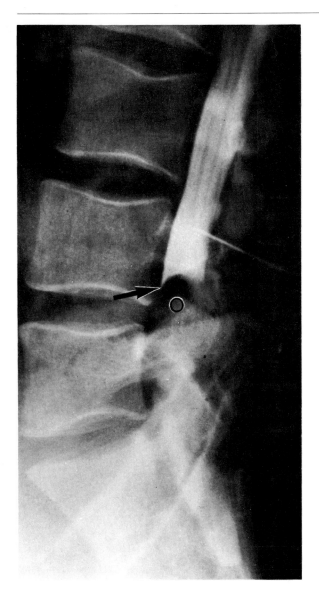

Figure 71

Lumbar neurinoma *(small circle)* hanging from the roots of the cauda equina. The tumor does not compress the anterior portion of the epidural space *(arrow)*. For this reason, lumbar phlebography was normal

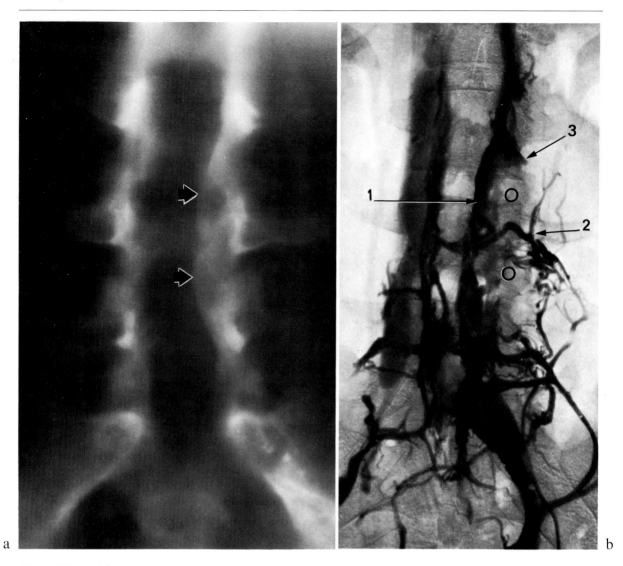

a

b

Figure 72 a and b

Lumbar neurinomas, Recklinghausen disease

a Air myelogram. AP projection. The intravertebral portion of a bilobulated neurinoma is demonstrated laterally on the left side *(arrows)* of the spinal canal
b Phlebogram. A molding of the epidural veins on the
  bilobulated neurinoma is observed. The absence of venous interruption is presumably explained by the fact
  that the tumor grew slowly during infancy and epidural
  veins adapted their shape around the tumor. If it had
  been a fast-growing tumor, the epidural veins would
  have been interrupted (see Fig. 74)
  1 Epidural vein medially displaced
  2 Extravertebral veins displaced and compressed by the
    extravertebral extension of the tumor *(small circles)*
  3 Molding of the extravertebral veins on the superior
    extremity of the tumor

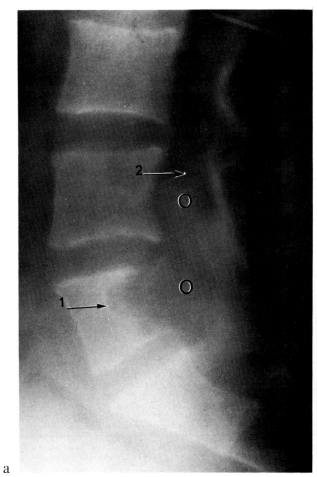

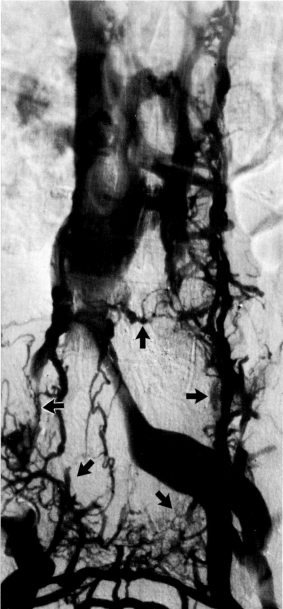

a

b

Figure 73 a and b

Tumor developed in the lumbosacral spinal canal

a Air myelogram. Lateral projection. The portion of the
   tumor developed in the spinal canal is demonstrated
   (small circle). There is erosion of the posterior wall
   of the vertebral body L5 in front of the tumor
   1 Erosion of the posterior wall of L5
   2 Superior extremity of the tumor

b Phlebogram. Interruption of the epidural veins in front
   of L5 and S1 and lateral displacement of the extravertebral veins demonstrating the exact extension of the tumor *(arrows)*

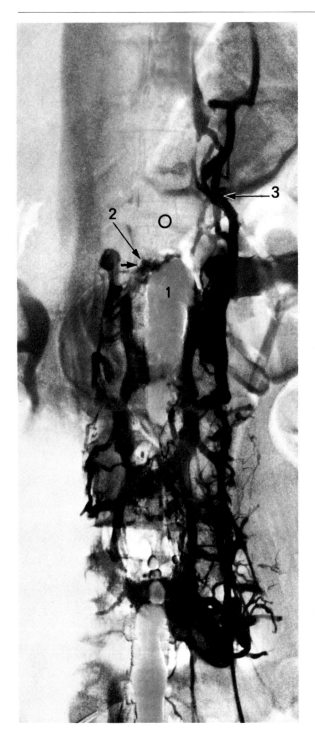

Figure 74

Tumor of the spinal cord *(circle)*. Interruption of the venous epidural flow in front of L1 that corresponds to the blockage of the contrast medium on the opaque myelogram *(horizontal arrow)*

1 Contrast medium (Duroliopaque)
2 Epidural vein interrupted in front of L1
3 Extravertebral veins bypassing the intravertebral obstacle

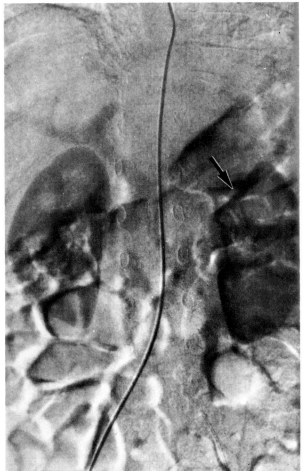

a

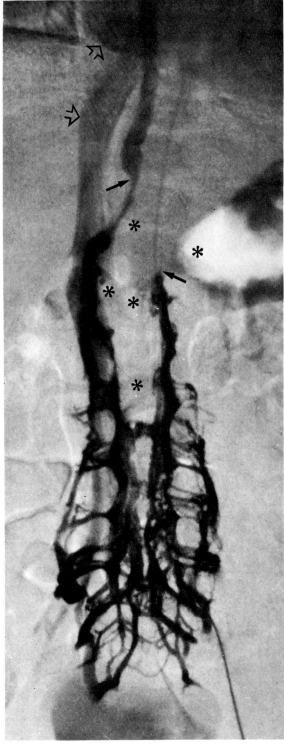

b

Figure 75 a and b

Ninemonth-old child; neuroblastoma with huge intravertebral extension

a Abdominal aortography. Late phase. A deformity of the medial side of the superior extremity of the left kidney is observed *(arrow)*

b Lumbar phlebography shows an interruption of the left epidural veins in front of T12 *(lower solid arrow)* that corresponds to the level of entry of the tumor in the spinal canal. The retrocorporeal anastomoses are interrupted by the tumor down to L2; the right extravertebral veins appear displaced in front of L1 by a small right extravertebral extension. Beyond the superior extremity of the tumor, the right epidural veins appear opacified again *(upper solid arrow)*. The localization of the tumor is indicated by *stars*. The inferior vena cava and the right auricle are also opacified *(open arrows)*. Surgery was performed according to information from pyelography, aortography, and phlebography which indicated the intra- and extravertebral extensions of the tumor

103

2.11. Stenosis of the Lumbar Canal

J. Théron and J. Moret

The treatment of lumbar stenosis requires accurate determination of the extent, location, and type of compression of the inside of the spinal canal. Clinical presentation is quite varied, and while the classic claudication described by VERBIEST [86] is often observed, lumbar neuralgia and sciatica may also be seen. The usual radiologic work-up involves plain film and tomographic study of the spine in conjunction with a contrast technique (opaque or air myelography, radiculography), the results of which often indicate laminectomy to decompress the canal. However, we think that more minor operations may often be chosen and still relieve the clinical syndrome; phlebography seems to provide evidence to support this view.

Two schematic anatomic types of lumbar stenosis can be recognized on phlebograms (Fig. 76), the results of which fit well with the classification established on plain films and radiculograms by BABIN, CAPESIUS, MAITROT [5] and WACKENHEIM [91]:

1. Concentric stenosis is due to an abnormal posterior arch of the vertebra with sagittalization of the articular facet interspace; this constitutes a small canal and phlebography shows a reduced distance separating the epidural veins of each side (Figs. 77, 78).

2. AP stenosis entails a narrowing of the lateral recessus of the canal but on phlebography does not show any change in the distance separating the epidural veins of each side (Figs. 79, 80, 81, 84).

Most of the so-called narrow canal syndromes correspond to the revelation of concentric or AP stenosis by the arising of an anterior (disc, vertebral body arthrosis) or posterior (articular facet arthrosis) lesion which, because of the stenosis of the canal, determines clinical symptoms more rapidly than in a normal canal.

Recognition on the phlebogram of the type of lumbar stenosis and of the exact extent of compression permits a better understanding of the anatomic lesions and consequently facilitates better treatment; intervention can often be more specific, for example, a single disc excision or a laminectomy limited to the extent of the compression determined from phlebography. Phlebography has shown that localized lesions can be overlooked by myelographic techniques which often shows only an extensive narrow canal; these lesions determine localized interruptions of the epidural veins on the phlebogram, and specific intervention may be preferred to an extensive laminectomy, and may nevertheless releive the syndrome (Fig. 79, 80).

While phlebography permits the accurate localization of the site of compression of the epidural space, it cannot differentiate between a compression arising from the anterior (Fig. 77) or the posterior side (Fig. 78) of the canal. Tomographic and myelographic techniques will then provide this information.

The phlebogram reflects precisely the degree of freedom or compression of the epidural space (Fig. 84). At most, phlebography can show extensive nonopacification of the epidural veins; this corresponds either to marked congenital concentric stenosis with no more "reserve capacity" [87] of the canal (Fig. 82) or to multiple disc lesions (Fig. 83). The first type is usually seen in young patients and the second, in elderly patients with a long history of pain. In both types lumbar puncture is difficult or impossible. In this case phlebography obviously cannot rule out a compression of the epidural space by a lesion growing in the canal, such as an extensive tumor, and complementary myelography is then performed, using a suboccipital approach, to provide information on the superior limit of the compression and sometimes shows the superior outline of a tumor.

Chronic compression of the epidural veins can cause a diminution of caliber of the extravertebral veins (Fig. 84b, c) because of the decreased venous exchanges between the intra- and extravertebral venous systems; catheterization of the extravertebral veins, in the course of phlebography, is, for this reason, often technically more difficult in stenosis of the lumbar canal.

The classification and description of lumbar stenosis seen above is deliberately schematic. The study of stenosis of the lumbar canal should be included in the general problem of the low back pain syndromes and it is rather frequent, on a phlebogram taken for sciatica or pure lumbar neuralgia, to observe a localized lesion (see Sects. 2.3 and 2.4) but also some degree of concentric stenosis, which has presumably accelerated the clinical onset (Fig. 85).

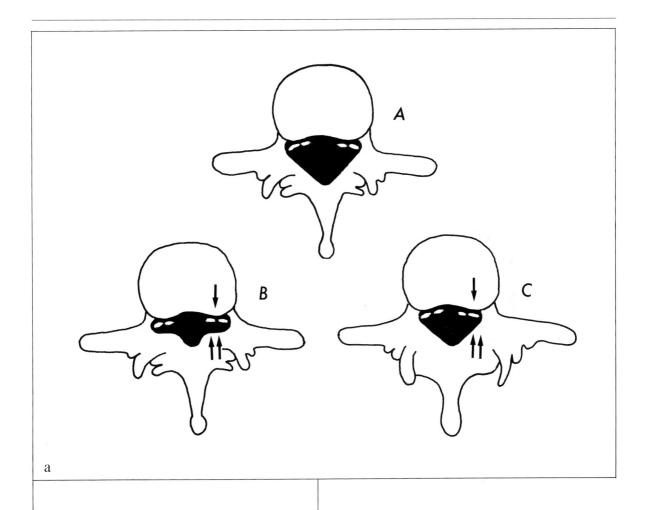

a

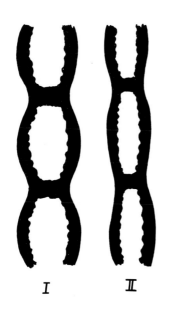

b

Figure 76 a and b

The two main types of stenosis of the lumbar canal and the corresponding pattern of the epidural veins

a Superior view of a normal lumbar canal (*A*), an AP stenosis (*B*) and a concentric stenosis (*C*). Most of the so-called narrow canal syndromes correspond to the revelation of concentric or AP stenosis by the arising of an anterior (disc, vertebral body arthrosis) (*arrow*) or posterior (articular facet arthrosis) (*double arrow*) lesion which, because of the stenosis of the canal, determines clinical symptoms more rapidly than in a normal canal

b Appearance of the epidural veins on an AP phlebogram

　I Normal distance between the epidural veins that can also be observed in AP stenosis [see (a), drawings *A* and *B*]

　II The distance between the epidural veins is reduced in concentric stenosis [see (a), drawing *C*]

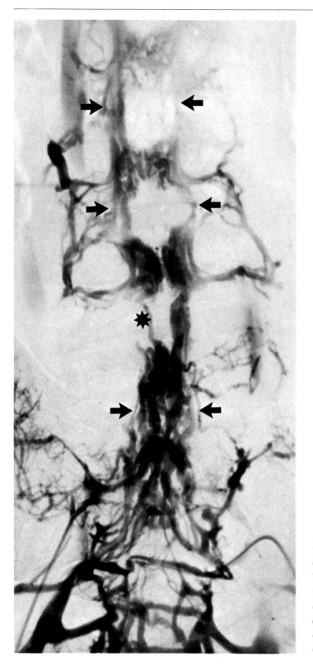

Figure 77

Concentric stenosis (see Fig. 76a, drawing *C*) revealed by a right disc herniation L4–L5. Note the reduced distance between the epidural veins in the inferior portion of the lumbar canal (space between the *arrows*). Right epidural veins are interrupted in front of the intervertebral disc L4–L5 *(star)*. Radiculography showed that the obstacle was anterior and was a disc herniation

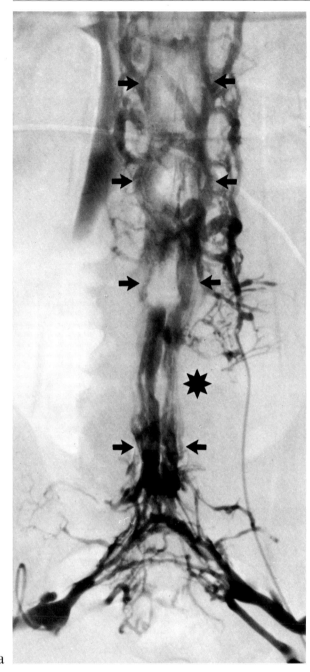

a

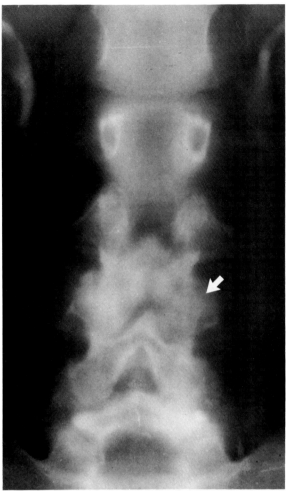

b

Figure 78a and b

Concentric stenosis (see Fig. 76a, drawing *C*) revealed by spondylosis of the articular facets

a Phlebogram: the distance between the epidural veins is markedly reduced in the inferior portion of the lumbar canal (space between the *arrows*). Left lateral epidural veins are interrupted in front of L4–L5 *(star)*. This interruption corresponds, in this case, to a spondylosis developed on hypertrophied articular facets. From the phlebogram alone it is not possible to determine whether the obstacle is anterior or posterior

b AP tomograms of the lumbar canal. There is hypertrophy of the articular facets, more marked on the left side, with superimposed spondylotic lesions *(arrow)*

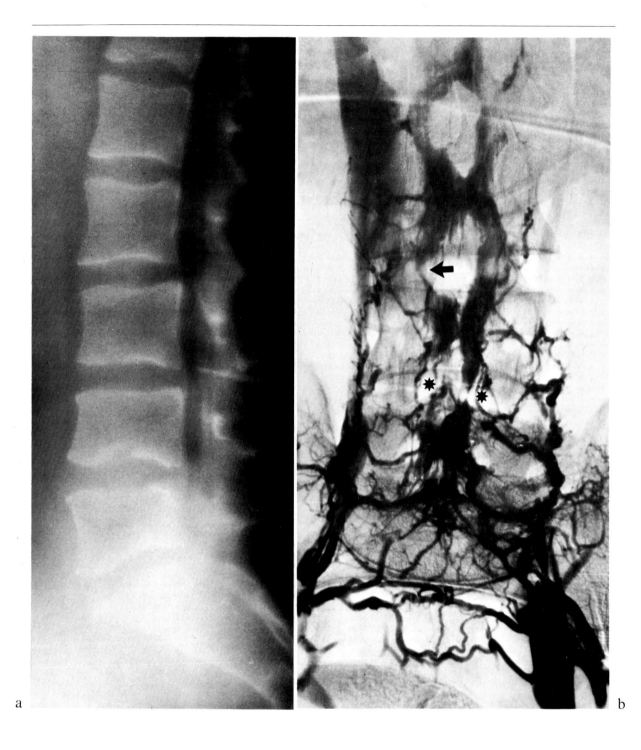

a

b

Figure 79 a and b

Anterior posterior lumbar stenosis revealed by disc lesions

a Air myelogram. The AP diameter of the canal is decreased up to L3. The inferior portion of the canal is poorly injected with air and it is not possible to demonstrate a disc lesion

b Phlebogram showing a bilateral interruption of the epidural veins *(stars)*, more marked on the right side, by a bilateral disc herniation. A minor interruption of the right epidural veins is also observed in front of L3–L4 *(arrow)*. The distance between the veins indicates AP stenosis (see Fig. 76)

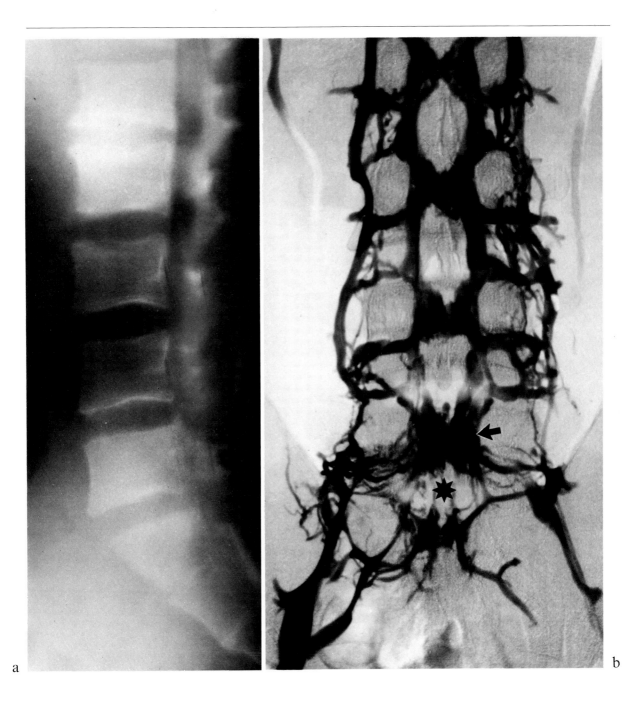

a   b

Figure 80 a and b

AP stenosis revealed by a disc lesion L5–S1

a Air myelogram. The AP diameter of the inferior portion of the lumbar canal is decreased up to L3. No disc lesion is observed in front of L5–S1

b Phlebogram. Interruption of the medial epidural veins due to disc lesion L5–S1 *(star)*. Retrocorporeal venous anastomoses in front of L5 are dilated *(arrow)*. The distance between the epidural veins indicates AP stenosis (see Fig. 76). L5–S1 disc excision led to the relief of the clinical syndrome

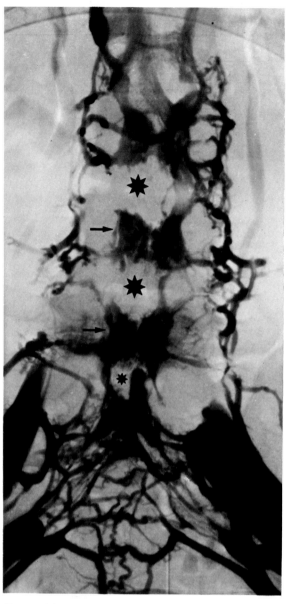

Figure 81

AP stenosis with multiple disc lesions. Phlebogram shows
a bilateral interruption of the epidural veins in front of
the inferior intervertebral discs *(stars)* with opacification
of the retrocorporeal anastomoses alone *(arrows)*. The
distance between the epidural veins indicates AP stenosis
(see Fig. 76)

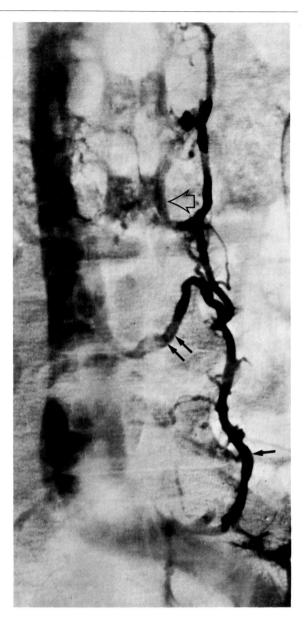

Figure 82

Extensive concentric lumbar stenosis. Young adult. Lumbar puncture could not be performed. Phlebography
shows nonfilling of the epidural veins in the inferior portion of the lumbar spinal canal. Injection of the left ascending lumbar vein *(arrow)* opacifies a hypertrophied
left lumbar vein *(double arrow)* diverting the venous blood
flow toward the inferior vena cava. Above L2 *(open arrow)* the epidural veins of the superior portion of the
lumbar canal are normally opacified. Phlebography, in
this case, can only indicate the extent of compression
of the lumbar epidural space; it cannot rule out a tumor.
In the present case other investigations showed that it
was a pure concentric stenosis with no superimposed disc
lesion or spondylosis of the articular facets. Noninjection
of the epidural veins reflects the absence of "reserve capacity" of the spinal canal

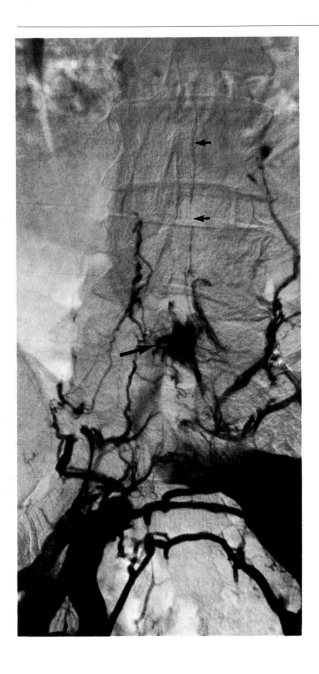

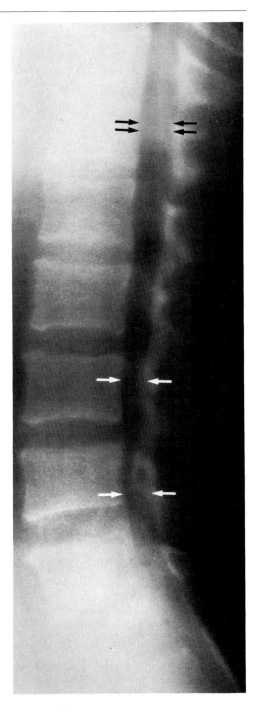

Figure 83

AP stenosis with multiple disc- and spondylotic lesions. Extensive compression of the epidural space in the inferior portion of the lumbar canal. Phlebography opacifies only a portion of the venous anastomosis in front of L4 *(arrow)*

This can be considered as a higher level of compression of the same mechanism demonstrated in Fig. 81. Here again, the nonfilling of the epidural veins does not permit a tumoral lesion to be ruled out on the strength of the phlebogram alone, and complementary myelography is necessary. Note also the retrograde filling of a radicular vein *(small arrows)*

Figure 84 a

Air myelogram. Marked diminution of the AP diameter in the inferior portion of the lumbar canal (space between the *arrows*). No obvious disc lesion is demonstrated

Figure 84 a–c

AP stenosis revealed by spondylotic lesions of the articular facets

113

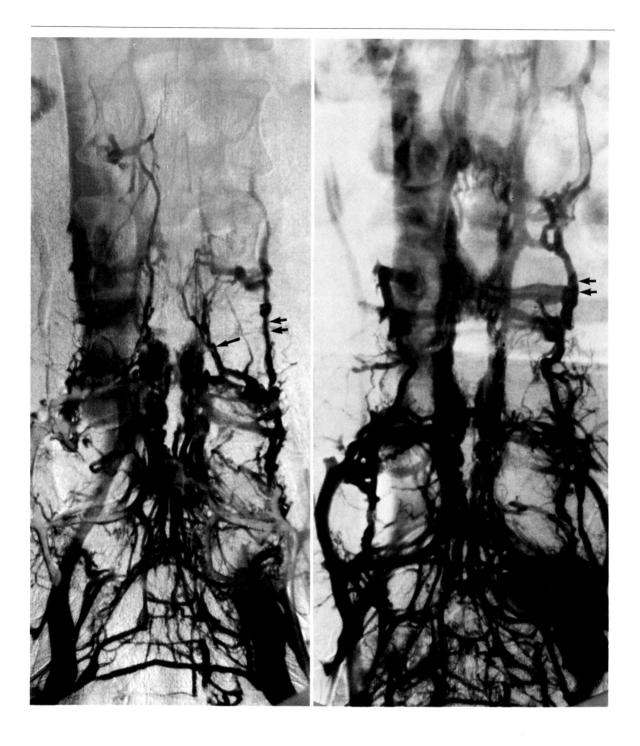

Figure 84 b

Lumbar phlebogram. The venous blood flow is almost completely interrupted in front of L3 *(arrow)*. The left ascending lumbar vein has a small caliber *(double arrow)*. At surgery: the laminas and posterior articular processes were portruding anteriorly and compressing the dural sac. No disc lesion was demonstrated. After extensive laminectomy the patient's condition was markedly improved

Figure 84 c

Second phlebography performed 6 months after surgery. Epidural veins are easily opacified all the way up. Diameter of the ascending lumbar vein is markedly increased; this can be explained by the increase of the venous exchanges between the intra- and extravertebral venous systems. Compare with (b)

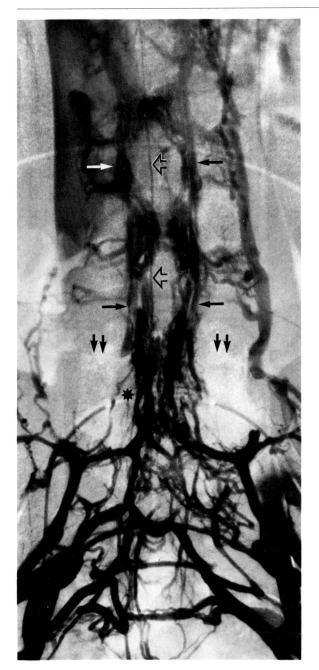

Figure 85

Lumbar neuralgia with no sciatic irradiation. Phlebogram shows an interruption of the right lateral epidural vein in front of L5–S1 due to disc herniation *(star)*. It also shows a certain degree of concentric stenosis of lumbar canal (distance between the *arrows*). In front of L5–S1 the veins of the lateral foramen are not filled on both sides *(double arrows)*; the same veins are normally injected at the superior disc levels. There is probably bilateral stenosis of the lateral foramen at L5–S1 on both sides. Note also the retrograde filling of a radicular vein *(open arrows)* draining into the epidural veins at the level of the disc lesion

Chapter 3

Cervical Phlebography

3.1. Technique, Complications, Indications, Anatomic Radiology

J. Théron and J. Moret

The first attempts to opacify cervical epidural veins were performed, as for the lumbar epidural veins, by puncture of the spinous process of a vertebra [77]. However, this technique did not provide regular filling of the epidural veins because of technical problems due to the thinness of the cervical spinous processes or because of the preferential filling of extravertebral veins.

In 1962, GREITZ et al. [46] described a new technique of cervical phlebography that consisted in the puncture of the 6th or 7th vertebral body via an anterolateral approach and injection of contrast medium into the spongy bone that permitted opacification of the epidural veins via the basivertebral vein. Opacification of the epidural cervical veins was more satisfactory compared to the difficulties encountered in the spinous process puncture technique. Other authors, in particular VOGELSANG [90], used it as a routine approach for the study of cervical pathology. Nevertheless the technique was not much used, presumably because of the rather frequent contrast medium extravasations and the irregular filling of epidural veins along the complete length of the cervical canal. For these reasons, far less attention has been paid in the literature to cervical phlebography than to lumbar phlebography.

In 1973, THERON and DJINDJIAN [82] described a new technique of cervical phlebography by catheterization of the vertebral vein on each side (Fig. 86). This vein was preferred to the anterior or posterior condyloid veins; these latter are also connected to the epidural veins, but injection into them does not provide good opacification with the same regularity.

Cervical phlebography by catheterization of the vertebral veins is generally a more difficult technique than lumbar phlebography and the experience of the angiographer determines the success of the procedure. When cervical phlebography is used in the work-up of cervicobrachial neuralgia, the procedure is performed under local anesthesia; the problem is then comparable to lumbar phlebography and usually consists in the diagnosis of disc lesions, as seen in Section 3.2. In the two other major indications for cervical phlebography, tumors and cervical myelopathy, cervical phlebography is often used in conjunction with spinal cord angiography; therefore phlebography is often performed at the same time as spinal cord angiography under general anesthesia.

3.1.1. Technique

When the procedure is performed under local anesthesia, a sedative premedication is administered to the patient (atropine, tranxene). The catheters (5 F, 90 cm length) are introduced into the femoral vein on each side using the Seldinger technique. The tips of the catheters are shaped with a slightly different curve on each side (Fig. 86b). Catheters are advanced in the inferior vena cava, the right auricle, the right or left subclavian vein, and then into the vertebral vein that is situated on the medial side of the internal jugular vein.

The angiographer cannot usually see the vertebral vein unless the catheter is already in it because of the normal venous flow descending from the vertebral plexus toward the subclavian vein. In practice, the vertebral vein is detected by the guide wire and the catheter is then pushed on the wire as high as possible into the vein; it is frequently possible to then introduce it into the transverse canal. Difficulties in catheterization are much more frequently encountered in elderly patients and also in patients with cervical myelopathy with cervical stenosis because chronic compression of epidural veins produces a diminution of the exchanges between extra and intravertebral venous systems and consequently, atrophy of the extravertebral veins (see also Sect. 2.11). In younger patients catheterization is fairly simple and unsuccessful procedures are exceptional.

Cervical epidural veins are studied on AP projection (Fig. 87); oblique anterior right and left projections that provide more information on the epidural veins situated on the side of rotation (Fig. 88) are also performed if necessary. Lateral projection is not usually performed because of the superimposition of the epidural veins and the extravertebral veins, which does not permit any precise radiologic analysis.

On each side 10 cc of contrast medium (Telebrix 30) is injected at a rate of 3 ml/s. During injection one film per second is taken for 10 s; the patient experiences little or no discomfort during injection. If the vertebral vein has not been catheterized on one side, the amount of contrast medium is doubled without modifying the rate of injection and the series is lengthened. Unilateral injection often provides satisfactory opacification of the epidural veins on both sides (Fig. 89); however, poor opacification or nonopacification of the contralateral epidural veins, when the vertebral vein is injected unilaterally, should not be considered as pathologic since, even in normal patients, unilateral injection does

not always provide bilateral opacification (Fig. 90). Limited nonopacification will only be considered pathologic if the veins situated above and below the nonopacified segment are well demonstrated. Catheterization of one or both anterior condyloid veins is now used only in cases of unsuccessful catheterization of the vertebral veins (Fig. 91).

3.1.2. Complications

Contrast medium extravasations can occur in the course of catheterization. The patient will then experience a temporary localized pain in the area of the venous effraction without any secondary consequences. The procedure can be continued a few minutes later. The frequency of this kind of complication depends on the angiographer's experience and will seldom occur once he or she is fully competent.

Infectious complications can arise if catheterization is not performed in strict sterile conditions; as is wellknown, this kind of complication is more likely to happen in venous than in arterial catheterization. Fortunately, none of the patients in our series of more than 300 cervical phlebographies experienced this kind of complication.

As with lumbar phlebography, thrombophlebitis can occur after cervical phlebography. In our series, only one patient presented with thrombophlebitis after surgery performed for a cervical disc herniation. Cervical phlebography is likely to be a predisposing factor for thrombophlebitis in patients who undergo surgery in the follow-up of the procedure. For this reason, we routinely inject 30–50 mg Heparin into one of the femoral veins at the beginning of the procedure and prefer not to use phlebography on patients who have a history of phlebitis. If surgery is indicated, the patient receives anti-inflammatory drugs (phenylbutazone). Since these precautionary measures have been taken, no more thrombophlebitis has been noted.

3.1.3. Indications

There are three major indications for cervical phlebography: cervicobrachial neuralgia, tumors, and cervical myelopathy. Presently it is in cervicobrachial neuralgia that phlebography is of the most immediate practical interest; it is performed under local anesthesia and surgery is often decided on the basis of the information provided by this technique alone. Opaque myelography (myelotomography) is performed only when phlebographic information does not seem significant enough. Correlation between phlebography and surgery is quite good (see Sect. 3.2).

For tumors, phlebography should usually be considered as a technique providing complementary information on a lesion of which the radiologic diagnosis is based on myelographic evidence. Performed concurrently with spinal-cord angiography, phlebography provides information on the extent of epidural vein compression and on any extravertebral extension of the tumor. Spinal cord angiography provides major information on tumor vascularization and on the relationships between the arterial branches supplying the spinal cord and the tumor; it also shows displacement of the vertebral artery by any extravertebral extension of the lesion. Phlebography cannot replace air- or opaque myelography, which provides the diagnosis in most cases, particularly in small posterior tumors which often are not recognized on the phlebogram because of the anterior position of the epidural veins in the spinal canal. However, phlebography can provide the diagnosis of small tumors developed in the lateral foramina and in metastatic epidural invasions before myelography (see Sect. 3.3).

In cervical myelopathy, phlebography should be considered as a technique for investigation of the level of compression of the epidural veins, the extent of then compression, and the relationships between the compressed area and the arterial branches supplying the spinal cord. This will be developed in Section 3.4. Here again, cervical phlebography cannot replace myelography and more particularly, opaque myelography (myelotomography).

Cervical phlebography is not indicated when spinal-cord arteriovenous malformation is suspected because this kind of lesion cannot be opacified when a venous approach is made (see Foreword and Historical Review by Professor R. DJINDJIAN).

Neither do we usually use phlebography in acute spinal trauma, where it could show an interruption of the epidural veins in front of a luxation or a fracture but would not provide information of practical therapeutic interest. Finally, a few attempts at phlebography in brachial plexus trauma have not shown any major venous modifications; but the procedures were performed a long time post-trauma.

3.1.4. Anatomic Radiology

In a normal patient, by bilateral injection of the vertebral vein, the cervical epidural veins are opacified from the occipital foramen down to the superior thoracic spine (Fig. 87). This opacification is obtained by retrograde filling of the normally descending venous flow. Opacification is frequently more extensive in the superior thoracic spine on the right than on the left side.

As was shown in the lumbar spine (Sect. 2.1), there is no posterior longitudinal epidural vein. All the longitudinal epidural veins are in the anterolateral angles of the spinal canal (Fig. 92). On a cervical phlebogram epidural veins present as a thick longitudinal venous strip where it is even more difficult than on a lumbar phlebogram, to differentiate the lateral from the medial vein (Fig. 87). In a few cases, however, this distinction is possible (Fig. 91). The epidural veins on each side are tied together by venous anastomosis situated behind each vertebral body; in the middle of these retrocorporeal anastomoses it is sometimes possible to distinguish the opacified basivertebral vein (Fig. 89). On each side of the basivertebral vein, it is often possible to observe a clear line on the venous opacity, which appears to represent the anterior branch of the nerve root (Fig. 89a). This is proven by its continuity with the image of the nerve root in the lateral foramen seen on some phlebograms (Fig. 90) and the stretching of the clear line in the rotations of the neck compared to its pattern on an AP projection (see Fig. 95, Sect. 3.2).

Cervical epidural veins are anastomosed with extravertebral veins superiorly and laterally, (Fig. 86 and 92). Superiorly, the cervical epidural veins are connected to the anterior condyloid vein via the suboccipital plexus. The anterior condyloid vein is connected to the inferior petrosal sinus and may be catheterized via the internal jugular vein (Fig. 91). Retrograde injection into the vertebral vein can frequently opacify the anterior condyloid vein with reflux of the contrast medium into the internal jugular vein (Fig. 88).

Laterally, the cervical epidural veins are connected to the vertebral plexus that surrounds the vertebral artery in the transverse canal; contrary to classic anatomic descriptions, the vertebral vein is individualized as a single vein only at its ending; the vertebral vein drains into the subclavian vein medial to the internal jugular vein (Figs. 86, 89, 91). The epidural veins are connected to the vertebral plexus via the lateral foramina plexuses that surround the corresponding nerve root at each vertebral level (Figs. 89, 90, 92). The vertebral plexus surrounds the vertebral artery and its negative image can frequently be observed on phlebograms (Figs. 87 and 88).

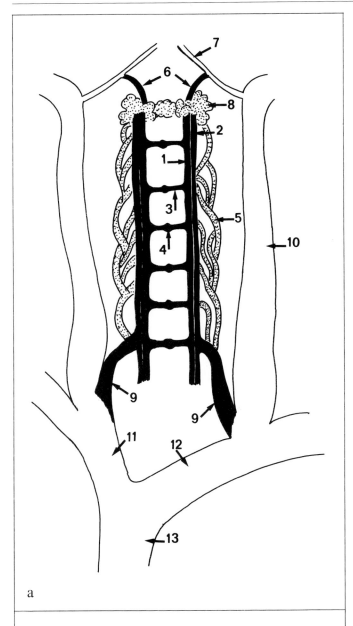

a

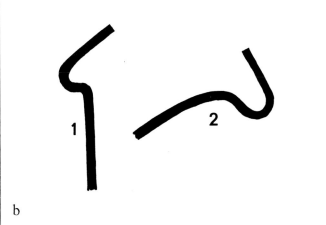

b

Figure 86

a Schematic drawing of the cervical epidural veins
  and their relationships with extravertebral veins
  1 Medial epidural vein
  2 Lateral epidural vein
  3 Retrocorporeal venous anastomosis
  4 Basivertebral vein
  5 Vertebral plexus surrounding the vertebral
    artery
  6 Anterior condyloid vein joining the inferior
    petrosal sinus to the suboccipital plexus and
    the epidural veins
  7 Inferior petrosal sinus
  8 Suboccipital plexus
  9 Vertebral vein
  10 Internal jugular vein
  11 Right subclavian vein
  12 Left subclavian vein
  13 Superior vena cava
b Tips of the catheters represented in position to
  investigate the vertebral vein in the subclavian
  veins on AP fluoroscopy
  1 Right side
  2 Left side

123

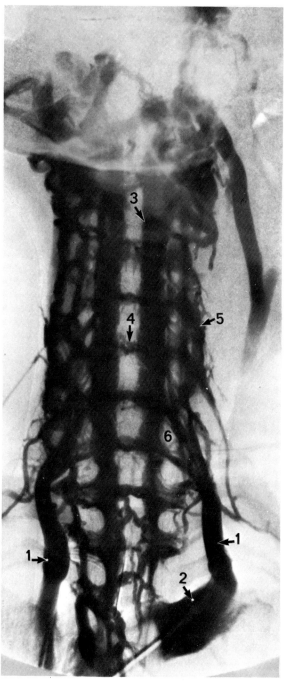

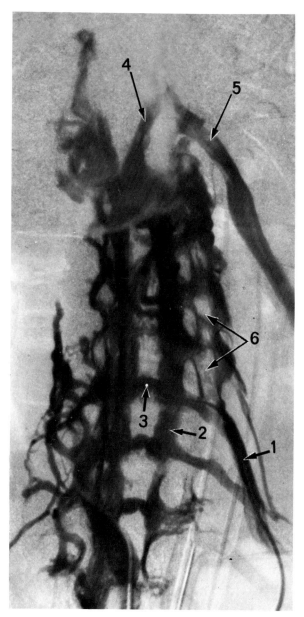

Figure 87

Normal cervical phlebogram. Bilateral catheterization of the vertebral vein. The intra- and extravertebral veins are opacified from the base of the skull to the superior thoracic area. *1* Vertebral vein. *2* Reflux into the left subclavian vein. *3* Medial and lateral epidural veins. In the cervical spine it is usually difficult in the thick longitudinal venous strip to distinguish the medial from the lateral epidural vein. *4* Retrocorporeal venous anastomosis. *5* Vertebral plexus surrounding the vertebral artery

Figure 88

Normal cervical phlebogram. Oblique right anterior projection. This projection usually permits better analysis of the epidural veins on the side of rotation of the body. The connection of the anterior condyloid vein with the suboccipital plexus is demonstrated and the filling of the internal jugular vein is observed. *1* Vertebral vein. *2* Left epidural veins. *3* Retrocorporeal venous anastomosis. *4* Left anterior condyloid vein. *5* Internal jugular vein. *6* Vertebral artery; its shape is recognizable within the vertebral plexus

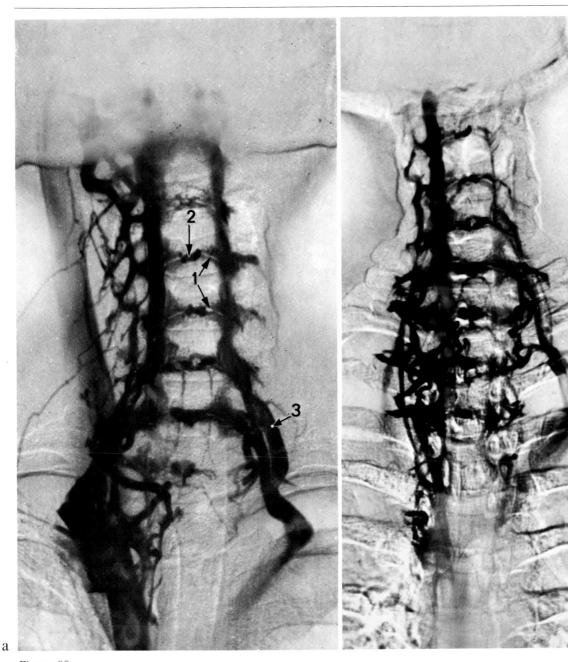

Figure 89

a Normal cervical phlebogram. Catheterization of the right vertebral vein. Opacification of epidural veins on both sides. Injection performed in the horizontal position
  1 Anterior branch of the nerve root surrounded by the epidural veins in front of each vertebral body (see Fig. 92)
  2 Basivertebral vein
b Same procedure, same injection performed in the vertical position. Note the absence of reflux into the internal jugular vein and the preferential filling of the superior thoracic epidural veins that were not opacified in the horizontal position (see Chap. 1)

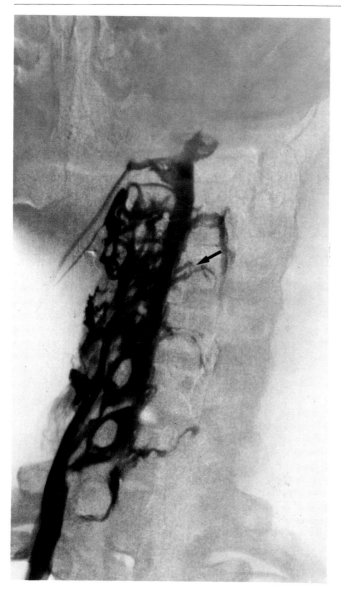

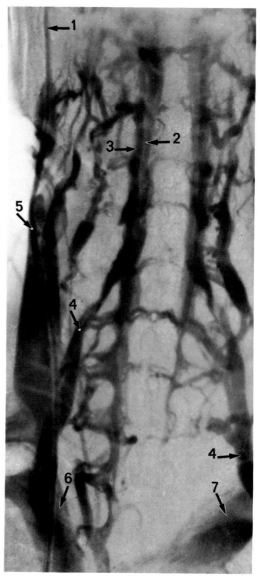

Figure 90

Normal cervical phlebogram obtained by catheterization of the right vertebral vein. Oblique left anterior projection. The nerve root surrounded by the veins can be followed in the spinal canal and the lateral foramen *(arrow)*

Figure 91

Normal cervical phlebogram obtained by catheterization of the right anterior condyloid vein. Good filling of the intra- and extravertebral veins. Actually, catheterization of this vein does not usually provide satisfactory opacification of the epidural veins but only of the extravertebral veins. On this phlebogram the medial and lateral epidural veins can be distinguished from each other

1 Catheter in the internal jugular vein
2 Medial epidural vein
3 Lateral epidural vein
4 Vertebral vein
5 Right internal jugular vein
6 Right subclavian vein
7 Left subclavian vein

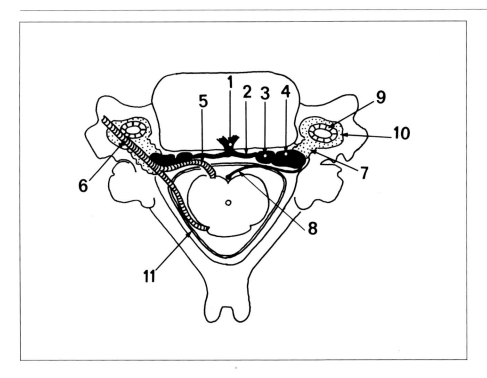

Figure 92

Schematic drawing of cervical canal as seen from above

1 Basivertebral vein
2 Venous retrocorporeal anastomosis uniting the longitudinal epidural veins
3 Medial epidural vein
4 Lateral epidural vein
5 Anterior branch of the cervical nerve root that can sometimes be recognized surrounded by the veins (see Figs. 89 and 90)

6 Cervical nerve root surrounded by the plexus of the lateral foramen
7 Plexus of the lateral foramen
8 Radicular vein draining the anterior spinal vein into the epidural veins and the plexus of the lateral foramen
9 Vertebral artery surrounded by the vertebral plexus
10 Vertebral plexus
11 Dura mater

3.2. Cervicobrachial Neuralgia

J. Théron, D. Chevalier and J. P. Houtteville

In most cases cervicobrachial neuralgia is due to the compression of a nerve root by a disc or a spondylotic formation. It is a common condition, but few cases need to be treated surgically. Surgery is now more simple when performed from an anterior approach, but to be effective it requires accurate preoperative localization of the lesion.

Up to now, 25 phlebographies have been performed for cervicobrachial neuralgia that persisted under medical treatment. The clinical level of the lesion was determined according to MURPHY's classic diagram [66] (see table), but the exact localization was sometimes difficult because the painful area seemed to involve more than one nerve root; also, one patient presented pure lateralized neck pain without any brachial radiation (case 24). Cervical phlebography was performed under local anesthesia by catheterization of the vertebral veins and was the first contrast procedure to be used on these patients. In 12 cases, phlebography was the only contrast technique used in the work-up of these patients; air myelography was performed in 6 cases, opaque myelography in 7 cases, and discography in 3 cases (see table).

3.2.1. Results

Cervical phlebography showed an interruption of the epidural veins in front of one intervertebral disc on one side in 18 cases (see table) (Figs. 93–96), on both sides in 3 cases (cases 6, 10, 17), and in front of two intervertebral discs in one case (case 9). In one case

epidural veins could not be opacified above C5 but were normally filled on the opposite side (case 14) (Fig. 97). Venous interruption was localized to the veins of the lateral foramen in two cases (cases 24, 25, Fig. 98); widening of the venous epidural strip above the pathologic interruption was observed in 3 cases (cases 5, 8, 10, Fig. 99), and in 4 cases, below the interruption (cases 3, 4, 7, 10) (Figs. 96 and 100). Marked hyperdensity of the venous retrocoporreal anastomosis was observed in 2 cases (cases 6 and 25) below (Fig. 101) or above (Fig. 98) the disc lesion.

The level of the disc lesion shown on the phlebogram corresponded to the clinical localization in 18 cases (see table); however, among these cases, clinically unilateral, the phlebogram showed bilateral interruption of the veins in 2 cases (cases 10, 17). In 14 cases surgery was performed on a disc that was clinically and phlebographically suspect, with good results in 12 cases and only partial regression of the neuralgia in 2 cases (cases 1, 25). In 6 cases, the interruption of the epidural veins on the phlebogram did not correspond to the clinical localization (see table); surgery was nevertheless performed at the disc level indicated on the phlebogram in 4 cases (cases 5, 8, 11, 13) with good results in each case. Finally, one patient (case 24) presented only a pain localized on the left side of the neck without brachial neuralgia; phlebography showed interruption of the veins of a left lateral foramen in front of one intervertebral disc, removal of which led to lasting relief of the pain.

Cervicobrachial neuralgias

Cases no.	Clinical signs	Phlebography	Air myelography	Opaque myelography	Discography	Surgery	Post-op. follow-up
1	C7 left	C6–C7 left	–	–	–	Disc excision C6–C7 without graft	Partial regression
2	C7 left	C6–C7 left	–	C6–C7 left	–	Disc excision C6–C7 without graft	Good
3	C6 right	C5–C6 right	–	–	–	–	–
4	C7 left	C5–C6 left	Small protrusion C5–C6 on the midline.	Small protrusion C5–C6. Slight enlargement of C6 left on oblique projection	–	Disc excision C5–C6 with graft	Good
5	C6 left	C5–C6 left	Posterior spondylotic formation C5–C6	–	–	Disc excision C5–C6 with resection osteophytes and graft	Good
6	C7 left	C5–C6 left	–	–	–	–	–
7	Post-traumatic C7, C8 left	C6–C7 left	Posterior spondylotic formation C5–C6	–	–	Disc excision C6–C7 and resection osteophytes without graft	Good
8	C6 left	C6–C7 left	–	–	–	Disc excision C5–C6 and C6–C7 with resection osteophytes	Good
9	C7 left	C5–C6 left C6–C7 left	–	C5–C6 left C6–C7 bilateral	–	Disc excision C5–C6, C6–C7 uncusectomy C6 with two grafts	Good
10	C6 left	C5–C6 bilateral, predominant on the left	–	–	–	Disc excision C5–C6 without graft	Good
11	C5 and C6 left	C4–C5 left	Midline protrusion C5–C6 Lateral protrusion C4–C5 left	–	–	Disc excision C4–C5 without graft and C5–C6 with resection osteophytes and graft	Good

12	Post-traumatic C7 or C8 left	C5–C6 left	–	–	–	–	–
13	C6 bilateral	C6–C7 left	–	–	–	Disc excision C6–C7 with resection osteophytes without graft	Good
14	C5 right	C5 right – no venous opacification on the right above C5	–	C3–C4 right C4–C5 right	–	–	–
15	C7 left	C6–C7 left	–	–	Perop. C6–C7 degenerated	Disc excision C6–C7 without graft	Good
16	C6 left	C6–C7 left	–	–	–	–	–
17	C6 left	C5–C6 bilateral	–	–	–	–	–
18	C7, C8 left	C6–C7 left	Osteophytes C6–C7; no premedullary air above	–	Perop. C6–C7 degenerated	Disc excision C6–C7 without graft	Good
19	C6 right	C5–C6 right	–	–	–	–	–
20	Post-traumatic C7 right	C6–C7 right	–	–	–	Disc excision C6–C7 with graft	Good
21	C7 left	C6–C7 left	–	–	–	Disc excision C6–C7 without graft	Good
22	C6 right	C5–C6 right	–	–	–	Disc excision C5–C6 with graft	Good
23	C6 left	C5–C6 left	–	C5–C6 left	–	Disc excision C6–C7 without graft	Good
24	Left cervicalgia	C6–C7 left	Normal	Normal	–	Disc excision C6–C7 without graft	Good
25	C7 left	C6–C7 left	–	Normal	–	Disc excision C6–C7 without graft	Partial regression

–: Not performed

Air myelography, performed on six patients, confirmed the phlebographic results in one case in showing a marked disc protrusion on lateral tomographic sections (case 11); in three cases a disco-osteophytic protrusion was seen on midline sections at a level corresponding to the phlebographic level (cases 4, 5, 18) (Fig. 99). In one case (case 7) (Fig. 100), the venous interruption observed on the phlebogram was situated one disc level lower than the disco-osteophytic protrusion shown on the air myelogram; surgery was nevertheless performed on the disc lesion demonstrated by phlebography with excellent postoperative results. In one case (case 24) the disc lesion compressed the nerve root in the lateral foramen and the air myelogram was normal.

Opaque myelography (Duroliopaque) confirmed the phlebographic results in 3 cases on the films taken with a vertical beam and the patient in the lateral decubitus position (cases 2, 9, 23). In one case (case 4) opaque myelography showed at the disc level indicated by phlebography (Fig. 96) only a minimal midline protrusion on the films taken with a horizontal beam and the patient in the prone position; oblique projection showed a slight enlargment of C6 nerve root. In two cases of compression of the nerve root in the lateral foramen, opaque myelography was normal (cases 24 and 25). In one case (case 14) opaque myelography showed two disc lesions that phlebography was not able to ascertain because a complete interruption of the venous flow was observed on one side with no opacification above C5; as has been already said, it is imperative to opacify the superior level of a venous interruption to be sure that nonopacification is definitely pathologic (Fig. 97).

In three cases, complementary discography was performed (cases 13, 15, 18) and showed a degenerated pattern of the injected nucleus (Fig. 102). Because these procedures were performed under general anesthesia, the reproduction of the neuralgia by injection into the disc could not be observed.

3.2.2. Discussion

In most cases, cervicobrachial neuralgia is secondary to cervical nerve root compression by a disc or a spondylotic formation. Surgery is not usually necessary, but in few cases, where neuralgia persists in spite of medical treatment or when the neuralgia is hyperalgic, surgery is indicated. The intervertebral disc is now usually removed using an anterior approach but, to be effective, will need precise preoperative localization of the intervertebral disc involved. Even more so than in the lumbar spine, clinical localization may be misleading and contrast-radiologic localization is necessary.

On the lateral tomographic sections, air myelography provides a good radiologic analysis of the midline and paramidline areas, but visualizes poorly the anterolateral angles of the spinal canal. Results can be misleading and the demonstration of a disco-osteophytic protrusion on a midline section does not imply that this lesion is responsible for the lateral compression of the nerve root (Fig. 100). This technique should in our opinion, be reserved for the study of the spinal-cord syndromes.

Opaque myelography is a harmless technique that can be very accurate when a sufficient amount of contrast medium is used and when mutliple projections are performed on the patient in various positions. The classic projection using a horizontal X-ray beam with the patient in the prone position is informative regarding only midline and paramidline lesions. For cervicobrachial neuralgia we prefer a technique using a vertical beam with the patient in lateral decubitus which, particularly when tomographic sections are performed, provides much more information on the anterolateral angles of the canal. Nevertheless, this technique cannot show a lesion growing in the lateral foramen. The other shortcoming of the technique is that it is necessary to introduce the contrast medium (Duroliopaque) into the subarachnoid spaces. This may be withdrawn or left in place, but resorption is very slow; this will be avoidable by the use of a water-soluble contrast medium (Metrizamide) once the tolerance problems have been solved.

Cervical phlebography performed by catheterization of the vertebral veins is a fairly easy technique when used in young patients; it can be technically more difficult in elderly patients because of the tortuosity of the extravertebral veins, comparable to arterial tortuosity at the same age. Phlebography is a harmless and almost painless technique that does not introduce any foreign substance into the subarachnoid spaces. The phlebographic signs observed in cervicobrachial neuralgia are comparable to those described for lumbar disc herniations; the basic sign is the interruption of the epidural veins that represent very good anatomic landmarks because of their position in the anterolateral angles of the spinal canal where a lesion can sometimes be overlooked on a myelogram. This is obviously also true for the lesions developed in the lateral foramen.

In our opinion, cervical phlebography seems to represent important progress in the radiologic work-up of young patients presenting cervicobrachial neuralgia. In most cases, by showing the exact level of the lesion, it provides enough information for surgery to be performed. When the information is not thought to be significant enough, complementary opaque myelography is then performed. In elderly patients, opaque myelography may be preferred as the first technique because of the frequent difficulties of catheterization of the vertebral veins; but it often shows multiple disc protrusions and the determination of which one is responsible for the present neuralgia is then difficult. Discography seems in this case to be of practical interest if the reproduction of neuralgia on injection of the contrast medium is interpreted as being more significant than the degenerative pattern of the nucleus, which is rather common, especially in elderly patients. It is rather in cases where this kind of indication is present that we would use discography in the work-up of cervicobrachial neuralgia. (We now use neuroleptanalgesia for discography; see Sect. 2.9.) Discography may also be very useful to confirm the results of phlebography in case of a disc lesion compressing a nerve root in a lateral foramen; it would then only be used on the disc level indicated by phlebography.

One last major point that has to be emphasized is that cervicobrachial neuralgia can also be secondary to a tumor in the spinal canal or to an epidural metastasis. Phlebography is not a very good technique for the work-up of spinal canal tumors but it can nevertheless be used as a technique complementary to spinal-cord angiography when the diagnosis has already been made using myelography (see Sect. 3.3). On the other hand, phlebography is a very accurate technique for the diagnosis of epidural metastasis because the veins are easily compressed and phlebography is positive even when the symptoms are not sufficiently developed to show up on myelography (see Fig. 105, Sect. 3.3).

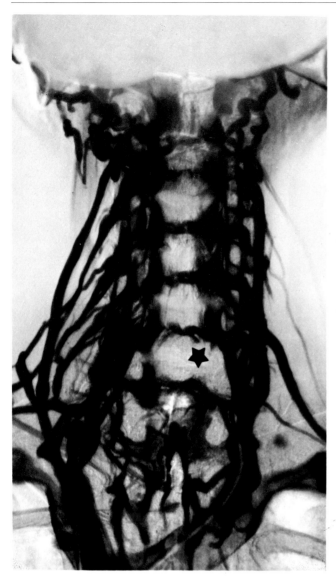

Figure 93

Left cervicobrachial neuralgia (see table, case 1). Cervical phlebogram. AP projection. Interruption of the epidural veins in front of C6–C7 on the left side by a disc herniation *(star);* good visualization of the superior and inferior limits of the interruption

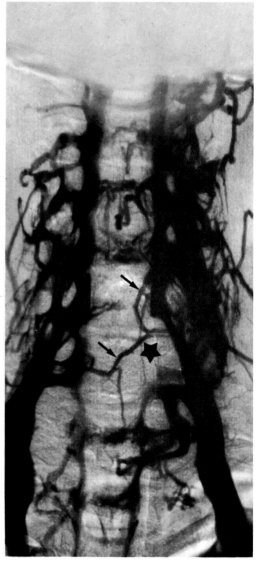

Figure 94

Left cervicobrachial neuralgia (see table, case 2). Cervical phlebogram. AP projection. Interruption of the left epidural veins in front of C6–C7 by a disc lesion *(star)*. Absence of opacification of the corresponding retrocorporeal anstomosis C7 and dilatation of a posterior vein *(arrows)* bypassing the obstacle

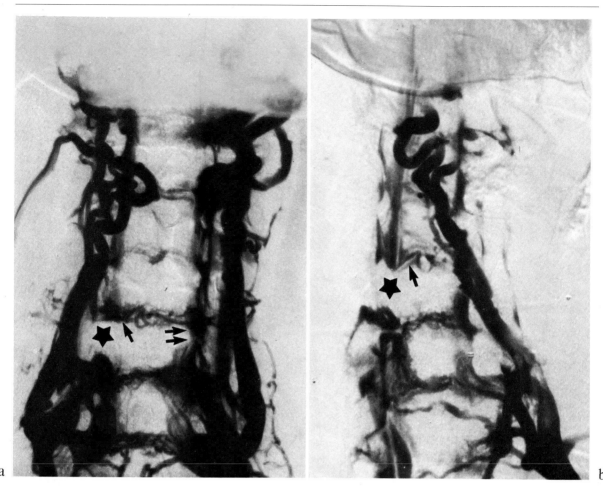

a

b

Figure 95a and b

Right cervicobrachial neuralgia (see table on p. 130, case 3)

a Cervical phlebogram. AP projection. Interruption of the right epidural veins in front of C5–C6 *(star)*. Minor compression *(double arrow)* of the contralateral veins. The nerve root (see Fig. 89) appears tortuous on this projection *(arrow)*

b Same procedure. Right oblique anterior projection. The nerve root appears stretched because of tension due to rotation of the neck in this position *(arrow)*

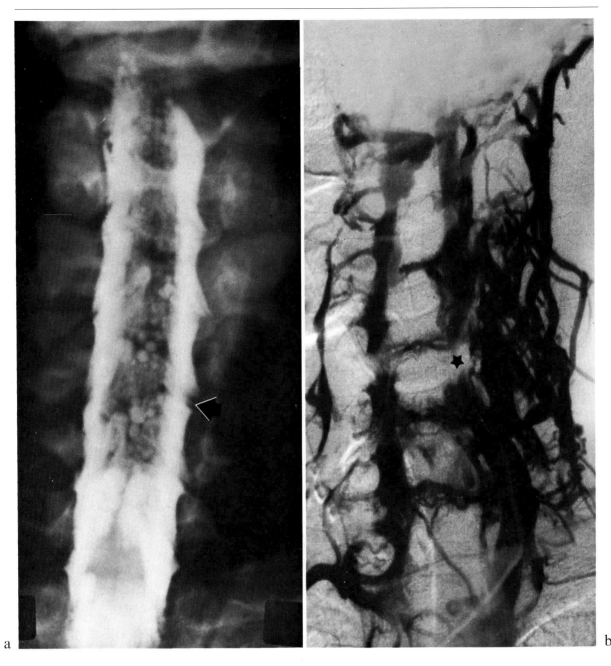

a

b

Figure 96a and b

Left cervicobrachial neuralgia (see table, case 4)

a Opaque myelogram (Duroliopaque). Right anterior oblique projection. Slight enlargement of C6 nerve root notch *(arrow)*. A small protrusion C5–C6 was observed on the midline on the lateral projection.

b Cervical phlebogram. Left anterior oblique projection. The left epidural veins and the veins of the lateral foramen (C5–C6) are interrupted by a lateral disc lesion *(star)*. As compared to myelography, phlebography provides, in this case, more convincing information on the disc level to be operated on.

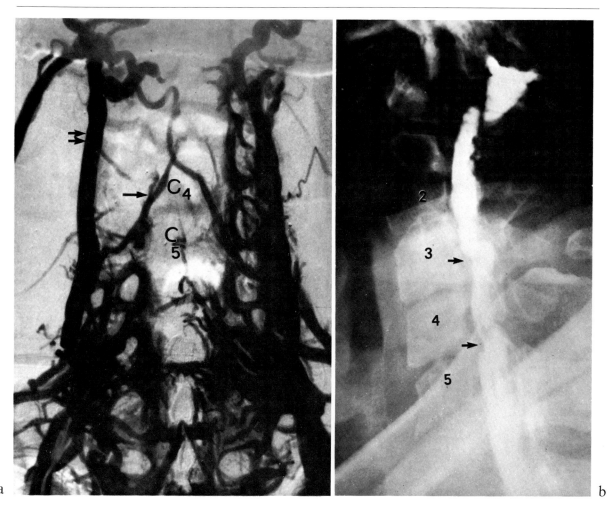

a

b

Figure 97a and b

Right cervicobrachial neuralgia (see table, case 14)

a Cervical phlebogram. AP projection. Right epidural veins are not filled above C4–C5 *(arrow)*. This interruption is pathologically significant because the extravertebral veins are opacified up to the base of the skull. However it is not possible by this technique alone to delimit the extension of compression accurately enough

b Opaque myelogram (Duroliopaque). Lateral projection, right lateral decubitus, vertical beam. This position allows satisfactory analysis of the lateral extremities of the spinal canal. Contrast medium is displaced posteriorly from C4–C5 intervertebral disc to the middle of the vertebral body C3 *(arrows)* due to disc lesions. This technique provides complementary information on the superior limit of the compression.

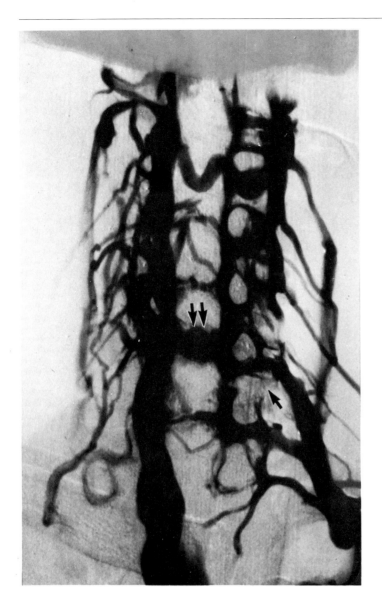

Figure 98

Left cervicobrachial neuralgia (see table, case 25). Right anterior oblique projection. There is no interruption of the left epidural veins. However massive opacification of C6 vertebral body *(double arrow)* and an interruption of the veins of the lateral foramen C6–C7 *(arrow)* are observed. Opaque myelogram was normal. The disc lesion was compressing the nerve root in the lateral foramen; this explains the normal pattern of the epidural veins and the absence of modification on the opaque myelogram

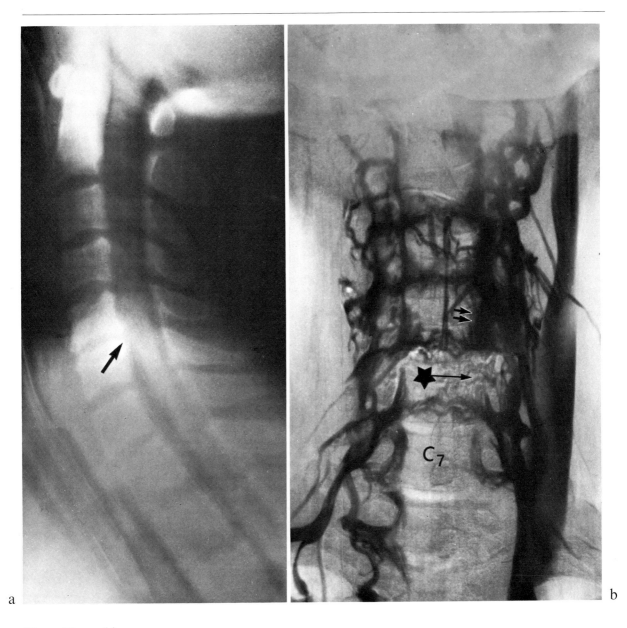

a

b

Figure 99a and b

Left cervicobrachial neuralgia (see table, case 5)

a Air myelogram. The intervertebral disc C5–C6 is narrowed; spondylotic lesions and disc bulging come into contact with the spinal cord. No air is demonstrated between the spinal cord and the vertebral bodies in the superior portion of the cervical canal

b Cervical phlebogram. AP projection. Epidural veins are interrupted on the left side in front of C5–C6 *(star)*. Note abnormal horizontal veins developed at the site of compression. Epidural veins appear dilated above the obstacle *(double arrow)*

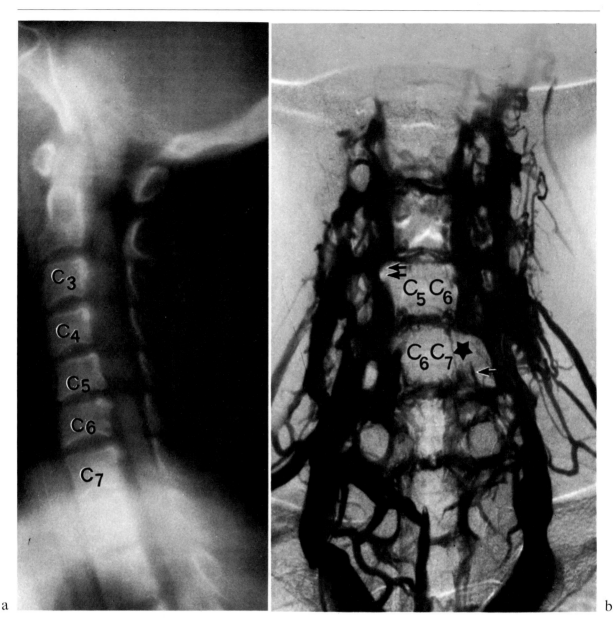

a   b

Figure 100a and b

Left cervicobrachial neuralgia (see table, case 7)

a Air myelogram. Intervertebral disc C5–C6 is narrowed with spondylotic spurs of the vertebral bodies coming into contact with the spinal cord. Minor spondylotic spurs are also developed on the posterosuperior aspect of C7 but no contact with the spinal cord is demonstrated

b Cervical phlebogram. AP projection. This procedure gives evidence that the cervicobrachial neuralgia was

actually due to a disc lesion C6–C7 on the left side *(star)*. The underlying epidural veins *(arrow)* are enlarged. Epidural veins in front of C5–C6 on the left side are normal (compare with air myelogram). There is a minor compression of the veins in front of C5–C6 on the right side *(double arrow)*. Disc excision of C6–C7 oriented by phlebography led to immediate and persisting relief of the neuralgia

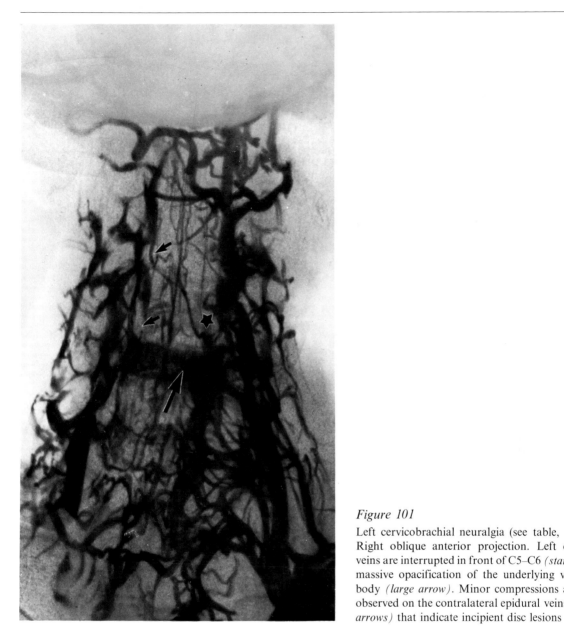

Figure 101

Left cervicobrachial neuralgia (see table, case 6).
Right oblique anterior projection. Left epidural
veins are interrupted in front of C5–C6 *(star)*. Note
massive opacification of the underlying vertebral
body *(large arrow)*. Minor compressions are also
observed on the contralateral epidural veins *(small
arrows)* that indicate incipient disc lesions

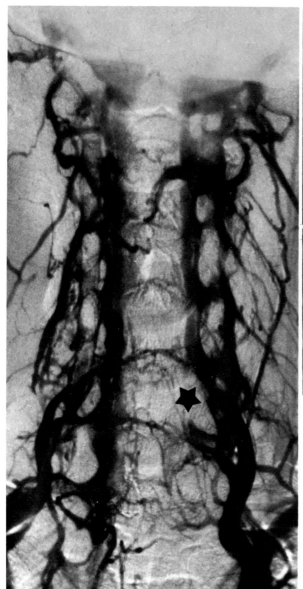

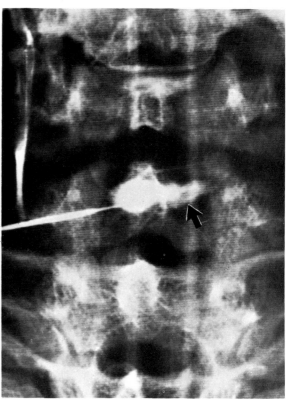

Figure 102a and b

Right cervicobrachial neuralgia (see table on p. 131, case 13)

a Cervical phlebogram. AP projection. Interruption of the epidural veins in front of C6–C7 on the left side *(star)*

b C6–C7 discogram. The nucleus is degenerated with leaking of contrast medium toward the left *(arrow)*

3.3. Tumors

J. Théron and J. Moret

Cervical phlebography should be considered as a technique that provides complementary anatomic information in the preoperative radiologic work-up of a tumor, which in most cases has already been diagnosed using myelography. Information from air or opaque myelograms is usually good concerning the intravertebral extent of the tumor but any extravertebral extension cannot be evaluated by this technique.

The preoperative radiologic work-up will also include tomograms of the cervical spine; if these show erosive modifactions of the vertebral bodies and an enlargement of one or several lateral foramina, it is very suggestive of an extravertebral extension of the lesion.

Spinal-cord angiography is, in our opinion, a major technique that provides complementary information by showing displacement of the vertebral artery by the extravertebral extension of a tumor (Fig. 103) and also permits precise localization of the arterial vascular supply to the spinal cord, to be taken into account during surgery. These radiculomedullary arteries and other branches arising from the vertebral or deep cervical arteries can also participate in the vascular supply of the tumor, the intra- and extravertebral outlines of which will then be well delimited.

We usually perform cervical phlebography concurrently with spinal-cord angiography under general anesthesia. If the tumor is large enough to compress the anterior portion of the epidural space, the epidural veins are compressed and appear interrupted on phlebography. Conversely, if a small tumor is located in the posterior side of the spinal canal and does not compress the anterior epidural space, epidural veins that are situated in the anterolateral angles of the canal (see Sect. 3.3) appear normal on phlebography. It could be basically the same in the case of a small anterior tumor growing on the midline of the canal between the two longitudinal epidural venous strips; however, we have not come across this kind of tumor.

Phlebography usually only confirms the results of myelography in the case of a tumor growing in the spinal canal but it provides the diagnosis in the case of small lesions growing in the lateral foramen that do not modify the inside of the spinal canal and do not significantly displace the vertebral artery (Fig. 104). Finally, phlebography is valuable in the evaluation of purely extravertebral lesions or of the extravertebral extension of a tumor of the canal, in showing the compression and displacement of the veins of the vertebral plexus in an area which can only be radiologically studied by tomography and vertebral angiography.

Epidural veins are easily compressed and are rapidly interrupted in metastatic lesions invading the epidural space even when myelography shows only minor modifications (Fig. 105) or none at all.

Intramedullary as well as extramedullary tumors modify epidural veins depending on the degree of compression of the anterior epidural space. Where large intramedullary tumors are involved, cervical epidural veins are not opacified because of the extensive compression of the epidural space (Fig. 106).

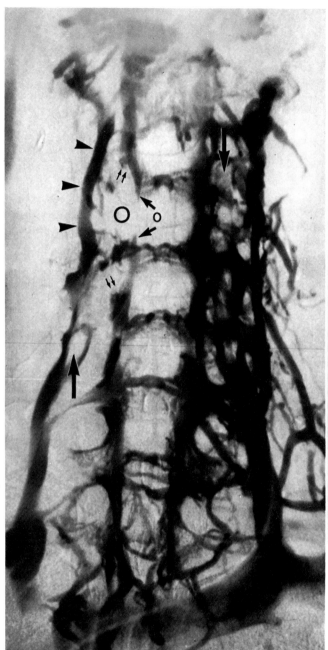

a

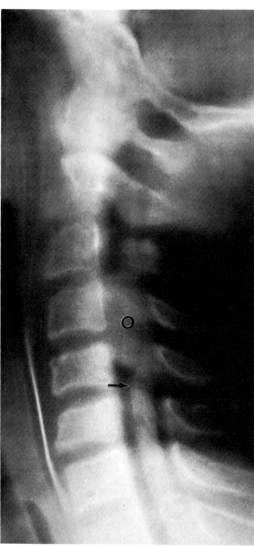

b

Figure 103 a–c
Hourglass neurinoma

a Cervical phlebogram. Intravertebral portion of the neurinoma *(small circle)* presents an extravertebral extension passing through the C5–C6 right lateral foramen. Interruption of the right epidural veins in front of C5–C6 *(arrows)*. Retrocorporeal venous anastomoses at the same level are not interrupted in spite of the position of the tumor coming into contact with the C4 vertebral body [see (b)]. Extravertebral extension of the tumor *(large circle)*, pushes the lateral extravertebral veins *(arrowheads)* and compresses the veins of the vertebral plexus *(small double arrows)*. Vertebral artery, outlined by the surrounding veins, cannot be followed in front of the extravertebral portion of the tumor *(lower vertical arrow)*. Compare with the picture of the vertebral artery surrounded by its plexus on the normal side *(upper vertical arrow)*

b Air myelogram showing the intravertebral portion of the tumor *(small circle)*. Absence of compression of the venous anastomosis in front of C4 on (a) can only be explained by the probable inclusion of the veins in the posterior wall of the vertebral body. Note also the posterior displacement of the underlying spinal cord *(arrow)*

144

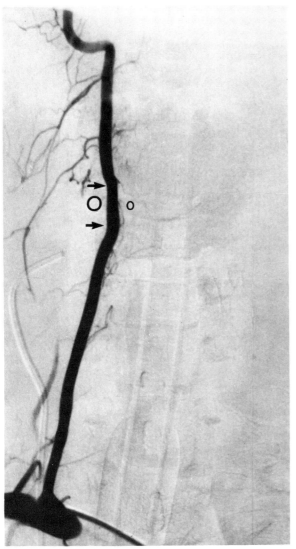

c

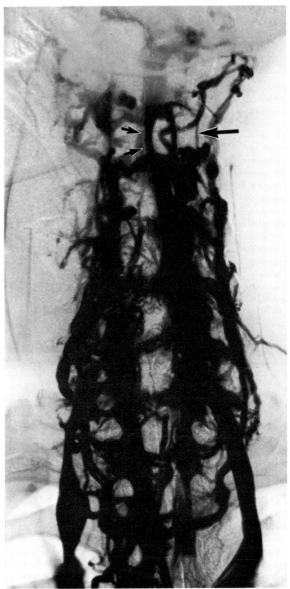

Figure 104

Recklinghausen disease. Small neurinoma located in the left lateral foramen C2–C3. On the plain films, in oblique projection the diameter of the lateral foramen was markedly increased. Cervical phlebogram: small neurinoma C2–C3 surrounded by the extravertebral veins *(arrow)*. Note slight medial displacement of the epidural veins in front of the tumor *(small arrows)*. Air myelogram was normal on lateral tomograms. Vertebral arteriography did not show any significant deformity

c Right vertebral arteriogram. Vertebral artery is medially displaced *(arrows)* by the extravertebral portion of the tumor *(large circle)*. Compare with the phlebogram (a). On the lateral projection, the vertebral artery was displaced anteriorly

145

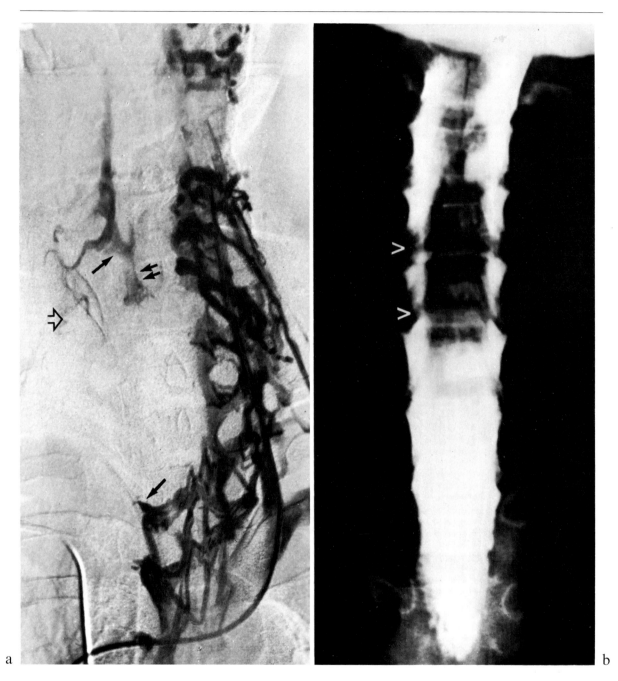

a   b

Figure 105 a and b

Right cervicobrachial neuralgia due to epidural metastasis
of a breast cancer operated upon 2 years previously

a Cervical phlebogram. Left oblique anterior projection.
  Right epidural veins are interrupted from C5–C6 *(upper
  arrow)* down to T3 *(lower arrow)*. Dilated abnormal
  veins are demonstrated *(double arrow)*. Right vertebral
  vein partially invaded by metastatic infiltration could
  not be catheterized *(open arrow)*

b Opaque myelogram. Minor right lateral notches are
  observed on the contrast column in the inferior portion
  of the cervical canal *(arrows)*; no slowing or halt in
  the progression of the *contrast* medium was observed
  on fluoroscopy. Epidural veins are very soft and will
  be the first components of the epidural space to be
  compressed in the case of metastatic invasion

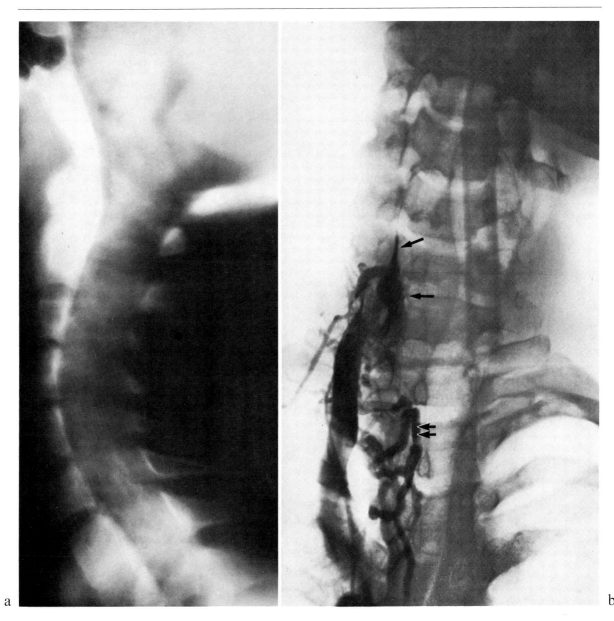

a

b

Figure 106a and b

Large intramedullary tumor (ependymoma)

a Air myelogram. Enlargement of the cervical spinal cord and the medulla

b Cervical phlebogram. Catheterization of the right vertebral vein. Contrast medium cannot opacify the epidural veins because of the compression of the epidural veins by the tumor; in spite of very selective catheterization of the vertebral vein the contrast medium stops at the entry of the spinal canal *(arrows)*. Diversion of the venous extravertebral blood flow is observed via the superior intercostal plexus *(double arrow)* toward the azygos vein

3.4. Cervical Myelopathy

J. Théron, D. Chevalier, J.P. Houtteville

Everybody has or will have spondylotic formations on the cervical spine. Fortunately, few people present with a "spondylotic" myelopathy, and those who do will not necessarily develop the most severe spondylotic formations of the spine. Therefore, one should avoid too mechanical a conception of the pathogeny of cervical myelopathy, which is often attributed only to the direct compression of the spinal cord by posterior spondylotic spurs of the vertebral bodies or by congenital stenosis of the cervical canal.

This exclusively mechanical pathogeny led, in France at least, to the performing of a great number of laminectomies intended to "make enough room" for the spinal cord and consequently alleviate the clinical symptoms. Laminectomies were usually planned according to the narrowness of the cervical canal as demonstrated on air myelograms, which showed how extensive the laminectomy should be [2]. In this purely mechanical conception, cervical phlebography may precisely show the freedom or compression of the anterior cervical epidural space (Figs. 107–109) but, being an indirect technique, it does not provide information on the cervical cord lesions.

For many years, other factors, meningeal, arterial, and venous, were suggested to try to explain this lack of parallelism between the narrowness of the cervical spinal canal, the extension of spondylotic lesions, and the appearance of myelopathy.

Induration and thickening of the cervical meninges observed on pathology specimens suggested a spinal cord stretching mechanism that was one of the arguments advanced in favor of section of the dentate ligament.

An arterial factor has also be suspected on the grounds of the topography of the spinal-cord lesions, which corresponds to the area of supply of the anterior spinal artery; ischemic pathogeny better explains the extent of the lesions that could not be explained by the simple localized mechanical compression of the spinal cord. However, if the compression of the anterior spinal artery seems logical considering its anterior situation close to the spondylotic spurs of the vertebral bodies, it is still difficult to understand why this artery is more severely damaged in some cases than in others and why the most severe spondylotic lesions do not automatically lead to myelopathy.

A lesion of the radiculomedullary arteries seems, in our opinion, a much more satisfactory explanation; these branches arise from the vertebral or the deep cervical arteries and enter the spinal canal at various levels. An "anatomic misfortune" could be imagined that makes a major and sometimes single radiculomedullary artery pass at the exact level of a lateral disc protrusion or a marked spondylotic formation of the uncus, consequently leading to spinal-cord ischemia; another patient having the same degenerative lesions might have the "anatomic good fortune" of not having a radiculomedullary artery passing at this level. This arterial factor in cervical myelopathy pathogeny can presumably be worsened by mechanical compression of the spinal cord, as seen above, and more particularly in hyperextension of the neck that directly compresses the anterior spinal artery.

Sometimes venous factor also seems to play a determining role in cervical myelopathy. This hypothesis, proposed by BRAIN, [10] was reinforced by the dilatation of the spinal veins sometimes observed in myelopathy, which has led some authors [1] to look for an obstacle on the extravertebral veins and particularly the subclavian and the internal jugular veins. Surgery has been performed to improve the caliber of these veins when stenosis was observed on phlebograms but, to our knowledge, the results have not yet been published. A more satisfactory argument for a venous factor is given by the retrograde filling of dilated spinal veins situated above a marked discospondylotic obstacle compressing the epidural veins (Fig. 110). As for the radiculomedullary arteries, a further "anatomic misfortune" could be imagined in which the radicular veins, draining the venous blood flow of the spinal cord, pass exactly at the level of a lateral disc protrusion or a spondylosis of the uncus; this compression would lead to dilatation of the veins and a lesion of the spinal cord (Fig. 111 a). Unlike the extravertebral veins, radiculomedullary veins can hardly bypass an obstacle; if there is a venous factor in the cervical myelopathy pathogeny it is, in our opinion, in the compression of the radiculomedullary veins. As with the arteries, this phenomenon can be increased by the direct compression of the anterior spinal vein in some movements of the neck, particularly hyperextension (Fig. 111 B).

It is likely that these various factors may interact and our radiologic work-up of cervical myelopathy is now set to analyze each of them. Presently we perform cervical phlebography concurrently with spinal-cord angiography under general anesthesia, complemented later by opaque myelography (myelotomography). Air myelography is much less used than at the beginning of our experience because opaque myelography seems, in our opinion, to provide more information when performed with the patient in lateral decubitus with a vertical X-ray beam and tomographic sections. This technique seems to give a better analysis of the anterolateral angles of the canal where radiculomedullary arteries and veins are compressed (Fig. 112 B).

Our present radiologic study of cervical myelopathy is based on a thorough investigation of arguments that could lead to excision of one or more discs and spondylotic lesions from an anterior approach. These arguments may be based on arterial, venous, or myelographic findings.

Arterial signs consist in the observation of one or more radiculomedullary arteries that enter the spinal canal at the exact level of a spine lesion demonstrated on a myelogram (Figs. 112, 113). Radiculomedullary arteries are usually dilated and sometimes distorted. This dilatation, already mentioned by others, seems to be a consequence of chronic ischemia and has also been observed in other conditions impairing the vascular supply of the spinal cord, such as trauma.

Venous signs are more complicated than we had thought in our early works on cervical phlebography. Phlebography provides information on the degree of freedom or compression of the epidural space but does not allow diagnosis of the lesions of the spinal cord itself. A congenitally "narrow" canal or a canal narrowed by multiple disc protrusions no longer has a "reserve capacity" [88] and the epidural veins are not opacified on the phlebogram (Fig. 107); in this case, phlebography is inadequate for localizing the pathologic lesion if we refer to the arterial conception seen above. Conversely, phlebography provides complementary information when the level of interrupted epidural veins corresponds not only to the lesion shown on the myelogram but also to the level of the radiculomedullary arteries (Figs. 112 and 113) or veins (Figs. 110 and 111).

On the basis of this radiologic work-up, seeking a convergence of arteriographic, phlebographic, and myelographic arguments for excision of one or more discs together with the spondylotic formations from an anterior approach, our early therapeutic results are encouraging. The postoperative results will be published when a sufficient number of cases have been followed up. We do think, however, that laminectomy should be mainly reserved for the few cases with severe posterior tracts symptoms; the other cases should be treated from an anterior approach.

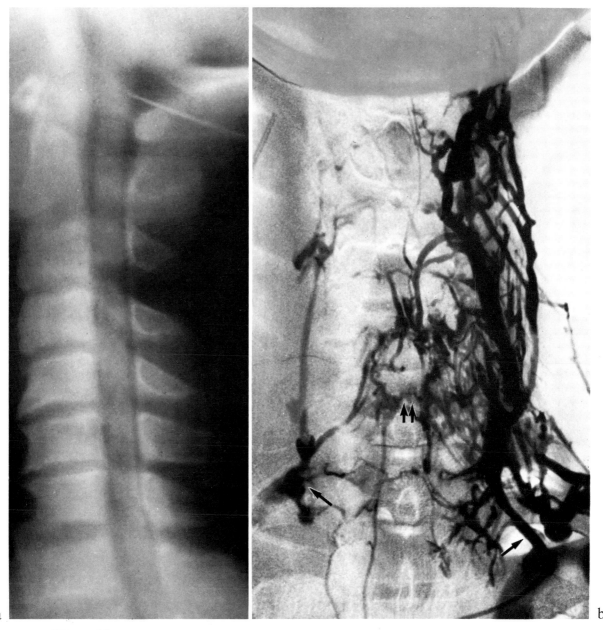

a

b

Figure 107a and b

Cervical myelopathy

a Air myelogram. Congenital stenosis of the spinal canal with no superimposed disc protrusion or vertebral spondylosis

b Cervical phlebogram. Catheterization of the left vertebral vein. Vertebral vein appears narrowed on both sides *(arrows)*. No opacification of the cervical epidural veins is obtained. Right vertebral vein is opacified via precorporeal venous anastomosis bypassing the inside of the spinal canal *(double arrow)*. This phlebographic pattern means that the cervical epidural space is compressed, but it does not give any information on the actual lesions of the spinal cord.

151

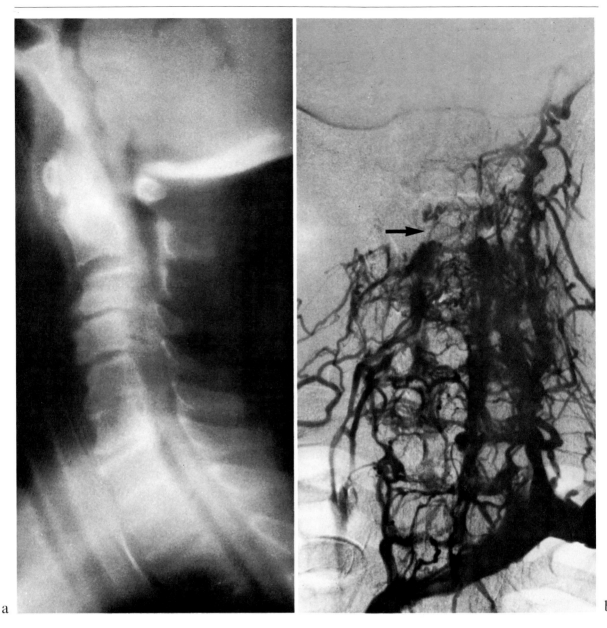

a   b

Figure 108 a and b

Cervical myelopathy

a Air myelogram. Marked stenosis of the superior half
  of the cervical canal with posterior subluxation C3–C4
b Cervical phlebogram. Catheterization of the left vertebral vein. Normal filling of the superior thoracic and
  inferior cervical epidural veins up to C4–C5 intervertebral disc *(arrow)* which shows the inferior limit of compression of the epidural space

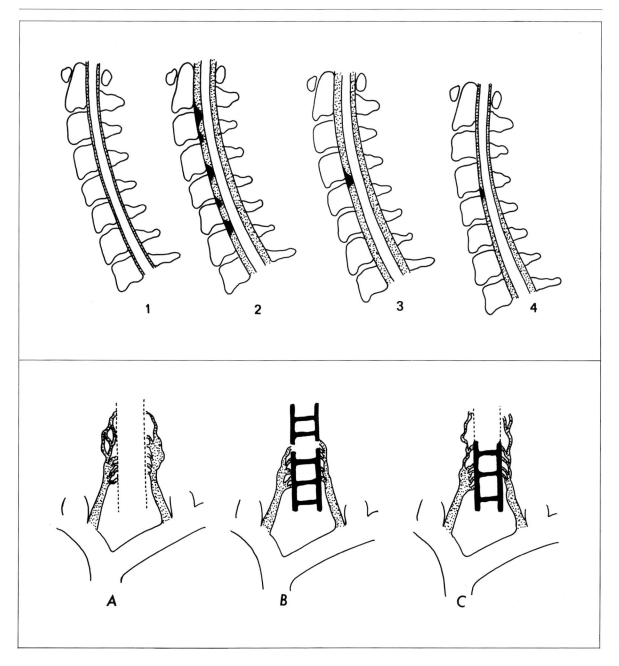

Figure 109

Diagram showing the various phlebographic pictures with the corresponding air myelogram pictures found in cervical myelopathy. This classification does not take into consideration the other nonmechanical factors that appear to be determinant in the pathogeny of cervical myelopathy as shown on the following figures.

1 Congenital stenosis without disc herniation
2 Multiple disc herniations
3 Single or few disc herniations

4 Stenosis in the upper portion of the cervical canal above a major disc herniation

A Nonfilling of the epidural veins that may correspond to types 1 or 2 of cervical canal
B Localized interruption of epidural veins that corresponds to type 3 cervical canal
C Filling of epidural veins in the inferior portion without filling in the superior portion of the cervical canal. Picture encountered in the type-4 of cervical canal

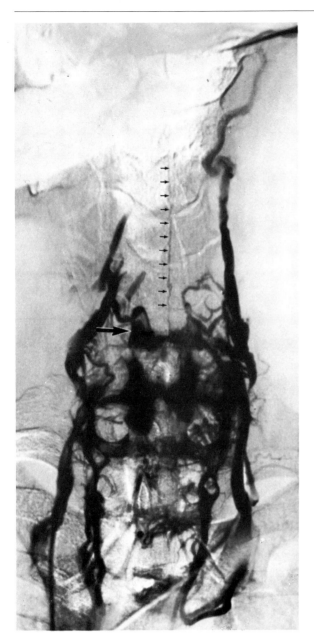

Figure 110
Cervical myelopathy
Bilateral catheterization of the vertebral vein. Good filling of the epidural veins in the inferior portion of the cervical canal. Interruption of the epidural veins in front of C5–C6 *(large horizontal arrow)*. Absence of opacification of the veins in the superior portion of the cervical canal. Air myelogram showed a type-4 cervical stenosis (see Fig. 109). A dilated spinal vein is observed on the phlebogram *(small arrows)*. The dilatation of this vein is presumably due to compression of the radicular vein that drains in front of the C5–C6 disc lesion (see also Fig. 92)

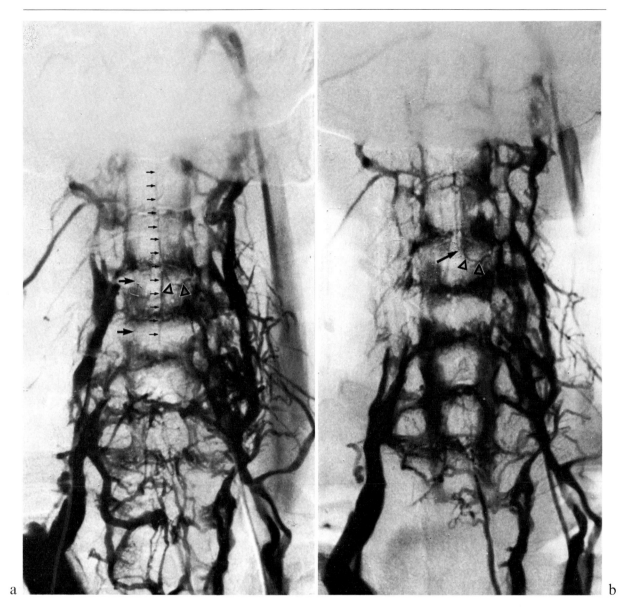

a   b

Figure 111a and b

Cervical myelopathy

a Cervical phlebogram. Epidural veins are interrupted in front of the C4–C5 and C5–C6 intervertebral discs *(large arrows)*. Dilated anterior spinal vein is observed on the midline *(small arrows)*. The corresponding radicular vein is also seen *(open arrowheads)*

b Same procedure. Injection with the neck hyperextended. Radicular vein is still opacified *(open arrowheads)* but the anterior spinal vein is now interrupted in front of C5–C6 *(arrow)*. Cases in Fig. 110 and 111 are intended to illustrate the venous factor, possibly heightened by hyperextension movements, that can be determinant alone or superimposed on mechanical factors in the pathogeny of cervical myelopathy

155

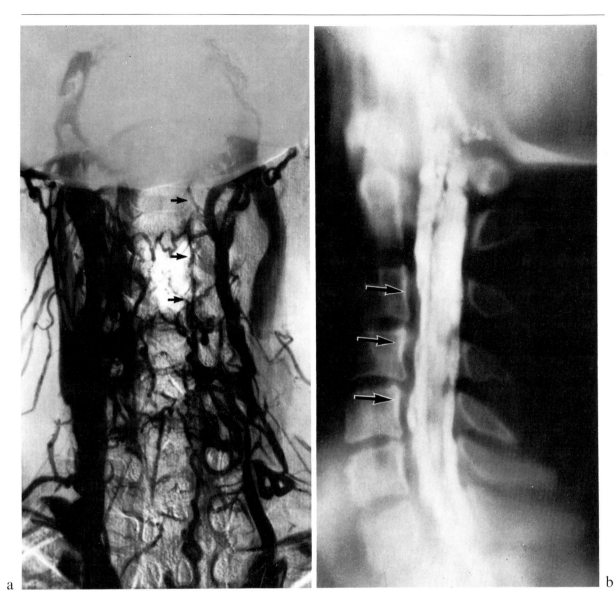

a

b

Figure 112a–c

Cervical myelopathy

a Cervical phlebogram. Good filling of epidural veins on the right side. On the left side, epidural veins are not filled above the C4–C5 intervertebral disc *(arrows)*

b Opaque myelogram (Duroliopaque). Myelotomography in lateral left position. Posterior displacement of the contrast medium in front of C3–C4 and C4–C5 discs *(arrows)*

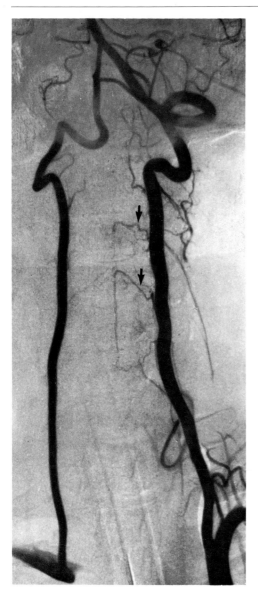

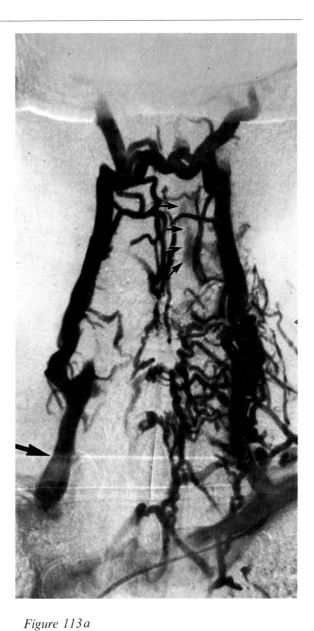

Figure 112c

Spinal arteriogram. Left vertebral injection that opacifies two radiculomedullary arteries passing through the C3–C4 and C4–C5 lateral foramina. Disc excision is decided upon on the joint evidence of phlebography, myelography, and arteriography. Intervention led to major and lasting improvement in the condition

Figure 113a

Cervical phlebogram. Catheterization of the left vertebral vein that opacifies only a short portion of epidural veins in the upper portion of the cervical canal *(small arrows)*. Diversion of the blood flow toward extravertebral veins and bypass of the inside of the cervical canal with contralateral opacification of the right vertebral vein *(arrow)*. Phlebography in this case can only indicate a compression of the epidural space in the lower portion of the cervical canal but does not provide more specific information

Figure 113a–c
Cervical myelopathy

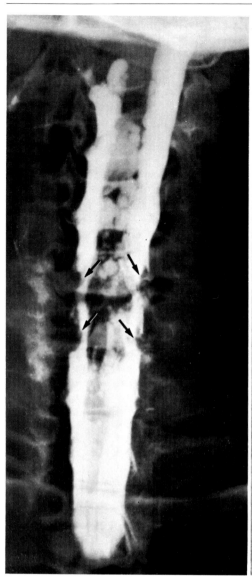

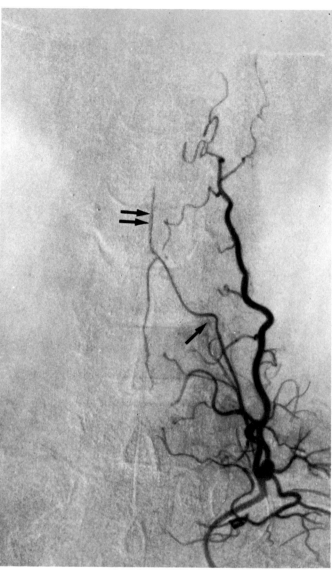

Figure 113b

Opaque myelogram (Duroliopaque). AP projection. Marked lateral notches are observed on both sides in front of C5–C6 and C6–C7 intervertebral discs *(arrows)*

Figure 113c

Spinal arteriogram. Injection of the left deep cervical artery. A dilated radiculomedullary artery arises from the deep cervical artery and passes through the C6–C7 left lateral foramen. This artery appears displaced superiorly by spondylosis of the C7 uncus *(arrow)*. No other supply of the anterior spinal artery *(double arrow)* is demonstrated by spinal cord angiography

Phlebography demonstrated only compression of the epidural space in the inferior portion of the cervical canal; opaque myelography showed compression of the inside of the spinal canal by C4–C5 and C6–C7 intervertebral disc lesions. Arteriography showed a single radiculomedullary artery supplying the cervical spinal cord that passed through C6–C7 left lateral foramen and was displaced by spondylosis of the C7 uncus. Convergence of signs oriented surgery toward the C5–C6 and C6–C7 intervertebral discs. Excision of these, associated with removal of spondylosis of C7 uncus, markedly and persistently improved the clinical condition. Cases of Figs. 112 and 113 intend to illustrate the arterial factor that seems to be most determinant in the pathogeny of cervical myelopathy

Bibliography

1. Aboulker, J., Aubin, M., Leriche, H.: Myélopathies par hypertension veineuse intra-rachidienne. Société de Neurochirurgie de Langue Française, 1971. Quoted by Lazorthes, G., Gouaze, A., Djindjian, R.: Vascularisation et Circulation de la Moelle Epinière, pp. 189–190. Paris: Masson et Cie. 1973
2. Aboulker, J., Metzger, J., David, M., Engel, P., Balivet, F.: Les myelopathies cervicales d'origine rachidienne. Neurochirurgie *11*, 87–198 (1965)
3. Ahlgren, P.: Longterm side effects after myelography with water-soluble Contrast media: Contrix, Conray Meglumin 282 and Dimer X. Neuroradiology *6*, 206–211 (1973)
4. Auquier, L., Rougerie, J., Siaud, J.R., Leparc, J.M.: Le curetage discal dans la lombalgie invétérée. Rev. Rhum. *44* (6), 375–382 (1977)
5. Babin, E., Capesius, P., Maitrot, D.: Signes radiologiques osseux des variétés morphologiques des canaux lombaires étroits. Ann. Radiol. *20* (5), 491–499 (1977)
6. Badgely, C.: The articular facets in relation to low-back pain and sciatic radiation. J. Bone Jt Surg. *23*, 481–96 (1941)
7. Baget, P.: Phlébographie lombo-sacrée par voie transépineuse. Etude anatomo-radiologique. Thèse, Paris 1961 (dactylographiée)
8. Batson, O.V.: The function of the vertebral veins and their role in the spread of metastases. Ann. Surg. *112*, 138–149 (1940)
9. Batson, O.V.: The vertebral vein system. Amer. J. Roentgenol. Radium Ther. Nucl. Med. *78*, 195–212 (1957)
10. Brain, R.: Some Aspects of Neurology of cervical spine (Crook-shank lecturer). J. Fac. Radiol. *8*, 74–91 (1956)
11. Breschet, G.: Recherches Anatomiques, Physiologiques et Pathologiques sur le Système Veineux. Paris: Villeret 1829
12. Bucheler, E., Dux, A.: Die direkte lumbale und vertebrale Venographie: Methodik, Indikation und Ergebnisse. Cesk. Roentgenol. *23*, 241 (1969)
13. Bucheler, E., Janson, R.: Combined catheter venography of the lumbar venous system and the inferior vena cava. Brit. J. Radiol. *46*, 655–661 (1973)
14. Bucheler, E., Dux, A., Venbrocks, H.P.: Die direkte vertebrale Venographie bei lumbalen Bandscheibenhernien. Fortschr. Roentgenol. *109*, 593–603 (1968)
15. Caron, J., Debrun, G.: Communication orale: Journée des Myélopathies cervicarthrosiques. Hôpital Tenon (Prof. Nick), Paris 8 Nov. 1974 Rev. Neurol. (to be published)
16. Caron, J.P., Hurth, M., Cophignon, J., Julian, H., Tayon, B.: Le traitement chirurgical des radiculopathies par cervicarthorse par abord antéro-latéral du rachis. A propos de vingt cas. Neurochirurgie, *16*, 221–240 (1970)
17. Castan, P., Bourbotte, G., Herail, J.P., Maurel, J.: Saccoradiculographies itératives et post opératoires. J. Neuroradiology *4* (1), 49–93 (1977)
18. Cauchoix, J., Bloch-Michel, H., Benoist, M., Chassaing, V.: Spondylolisthésis dégénératif. La Nouv. Presse Méd. *5* (9), 561–564 (1976)
19. Chakravorty, B.G.: Arterial supply of the cervical spinal cord and its relation to the cervical myelopathy in spondylosis, pp. 232–251. Royal College of Surgeons of England (1967)
20. Cloward, R.B.: The anterior approach for removal of ruptured cervical disks. J. Neurosurg. *15*, 602–617 (1958)
21. Debeyre, J., Delforges, P.: Arthrodèse vertébrale intersomatique. Rev. Chir. Orthop. *45*, 885–894 (1959)
22. Dehaene, I.: Diagnostic des hernies discales cervicales par la discographie. Acta Neurol. Belg. *72*, 318 (1972)
23. De Palma, A.F., Rothman, R.H.: The Intervertebral Disc. Philadelphia: Saunders Co. 1970
24. Dilenge, D., Perey, B.: Le drainage veineux méningorachidien dans l'hémodynamique cérébrale. Journées internationales sur la circulation cérébrale, Toulouse, 1972. Rev. Med. Toulouse, Suppl. *1973*, 43–49
25. Dilenge, D., Perey, B.: An angiographic study of the meningorachidian venous system. Radiology *108*, 333–337 (1973)
26. Dilenge, D., Geraud, G., Perey, B.: Recent physiological studies on the vertebral venous plexus. Atti del IX Congresso Internationale di Angiologia, Vol. IV (1976)
27. Dilenge, D., Perey, B., Geraud, G., Nutik, S.: Angiographic demonstration of the cervical vertebral venous plexus in man. J. Can. Assoc. Radiol. *26*, (2), 77–81 (1975)
28. Djindjian, R., Dorland, P.: Phlébographie rachidienne par voie transépineuse. Ann. Radiol. *3* (7/8), 449–468 (1960)
29. Djindjian, R., Dorland, P., Baget, P.: La phlébographie vertébro-rachidienne lombaire. Presse Med. Suppl. I, *73* (4), 131 (1965)

30. Djindjian, R., Hurth, M., Houdart, R.: L'angiographie de la Moelle Epinière, Paris: Masson et Cie. 1970

31. Djindjian, R., Pansini, A., Dorland, P.: Phlébographie vertébro-rachidienne par voie transépineuse. Acta Radiol. 689–701 (1963)

32. Drasin, G.F., Daffner, R.H., Sexton, R.F., Cheatham, W.C.: Epidural venography: diagnosis of herniated lumbar intervertebral disc and other disease of the epidural space. Amer. J. Roentgenol. Radium Ther. Nucl. Med. *126*, 1010–1016 (1976)

33. Ducuing, Guilhem, Engalbert, Poulhes, Baux: La phlébographie du pelvis par voie trans-osseuse pubienne. Lyon Chir. *46*, 393–404 (1951)

34. Epstein, B.S.: Low back pain associated with varices of the epidural veins simulating herniation of the nucleus pulposus. Amer. J. Roentgenol. *57*, 736 (1947)

35. Epstein, B.S., Epstein, J.A., Jones, M.D.: Lumbar spondylolisthesis with isthmic defects. Radiol. Clin. N. Amer. *XV* (2), 261–273 (1977)

36. Epstein, B.S., Epstein, J.A., Jones, M.D.: Degeneratrive spondylolisthesis with an intact neural arch. Radiol. Clin. N. Amer. *XV* (2), 275–287 (1977)

37. Epstein, H.M., Linde, H.W., Crampton, A.R.: The vertebral venous plexus as a major cerebral venous outflow tract. Anesthesiology *32*, 332–337 (1970)

38. Finney, L.A., Gargano, F.P., Buermann, A.: Intraosseous vertebral venography in diagnosis of lumbar disc disease. Amer. J. Roentgenol. *92*, 1282–1292 (1964)

39. Fischgold, H., Adam, H., Ecoiffier, J., Piequet, J.: Opacification des plexus rachidiens et des veines azygos par voie osseuse. J. Radiol. Electrol. Med. Nucl. *33*, 37 (1952)

40. Fischgold, H., Clement, J.C., Talairach, J., Ecoiffier, J.: Opacification des systèmes veineux rachidiens et crâniens par voie osseuse. Presse Méd. *60*, 599–601 (1952)

41. Gargano, F.P., Meyer, J.D., Sheldon, J.J.: Transfemoral ascending lumbar catheterization of the epidural veins in lumbar disc disease. Radiology *III*, 329–336 (1974)

42. Geraud, G., Viguie, E., Arsenault, A., Nutik, S., Perey, B., Dilenge, D.: Effets de l'hyperpression thoracique sur la circulation cérébrale du singe en fonction de la position du corps, couchée ou debout. Acta Radiol. Suppl. *347*, 87–98 (1975)

43. Gershater, R., Holgate, R.C.: Lumbar epidural venography in the diagnosis of disc herniations. Amer. J. Roentgenol. *126*, 992–1002 (1976)

44. Gillot, C.L., Singer, B.: La veine en L_2. Arch. Anat. Pathol. *22* (4), 307–311 (1974)

45. Ginestie, J.F., Fassio, B., Connes, H., Buscayret, C., Castan, P.H., Vidal, J.: L'Apport des explorations modernes dans l'etude des colonnes postérieures du rachis lombaire. Communication getroa (1976)

46. Greitz, T., Lilliequist, B., Muller, R.: Cervical vertebral phlebography. Acta Radiol. *57*, 353–365 (1962)

47. Guerinel, G., Artignan, P., Richelme, H.: Les veines lombaires et la veine lombaire ascendante. Travaux du lab. D'Anatomie (Marseille) *1965*, 43–45

48. Helander, C.B., Lindbom, A.: Sacrolumbar venography. Acta Radiol. *44*, 397–409 (1955)

49. Hughes, J.T., Brownell, B.: Cervical spondylosis complicated by anterior spinal artery thrombosis. Neurology *14*, 1073 (1964)

50. Isherwood, I.: Spinal intra-osseous venography. Clin. Radiol. *13*, 73–82 (1962)

51. Jones, R.A.C., Thompson, J.L.G.: The narrow lumbar canal. A clinical and radiological review. J. Bone Jt Surg. *50*B, 595–605 (1968)

52. Kahn, E.A.: The role of the dentate ligament in spinal cord compression and the syndrome of latent sclerosis. J. Neurosurg. *4*, 191 (1947)

53. Komminoth, R., Woringer, E., Philippi, R.: Megacul de sac dural. Etude clinique de 10 cas. Neurochirurgie *14* (5), 607–616 (1968)

54. Larde, D.: Les Veines Epidurales Lombo-Sacrées. Etude anatomique et radiologique. Intérêt de la phlébographie lombaire dans le diagnostic des discopathies. Thèse Med., Nancy (1977)

55. Lazorthes, G., Gouaze, A., Djindjian, R.: Vascularisation et Circulation de la Moelle Epinière. Paris: Masson 1973

56. Leger, L., Masse, Ph.: La phlébographie transspongio-calcanéenne. Presse Méd. *59*, 1560–1561 (1951)

57. Lepage, J.R.: Transfemoral ascending lumbar catheterization of the epidural veins. Radiology *III*, 337–339 (1974)

58. Mac Nab, I.S.T., Louis, E., Grabias, S.: Selective ascending lumbo-sacral venography in the assessment of lumbar-disc herniation. J. Bone Jt Surg. *58* (8), 1093–1098 (1976)

59. Mair, W.G.P., Druckman, R.: The pathology of spinal cord lésions and their relation to the clinical features in protrusion of cervical intervertebral discs. Brain *76*, 70–91 (1953)

60. Mascozzi, Messinetti, Saracca, Colombate: Phlebografia Vertebrale Transsomatica, Rome: Edit. Med. Sci. 1959

61. Maslow, G.S., Rothman, R.: The Facet Joints: Another Look. Bull N.Y. Acad. Med. *51* (11), 1294–1311 (1975)

62. Massare, C., Bernageau, G.: Le spondylolisthésis lombo sacré; examens radiologiques. Rev. Chir. Orthop. *57* (1), 110–114 (1971)

63. Massare, C., Bard, M., Benoist, M., Cauchoix, J., Bloch-Michel, H.: Renseignements fournis par la discographie lombaire pour le diagnostic et le traitement chirurgical des discopathies douloureuses lombaires et lombo-sacrées. Rev. Rhum. *41*, 113–122 (1974)

64. Miller, M.H., Handel, S.F., Coan, J.D.: Transfemoral lumbar epidural venography. Amer. J. Roentgenol. *126*, 1003–1009 (1976)

65. Moret, J., Vignaud, J., Doyon, D.: Techniques d'opacification des plexus veineux intra-rachidiens lombaires. J. Radiol. Electrol. *57* (6–7), 553–560 (1976)

66. Murphy, F., James, M.D., Simmon, D.S.: Ruptured cervical disc experience with 250 cases. Amer. Surg. *32* (2), 83 (1966)

67. Payne, E.E., Spillane, J.D.: The cervical spine. An anatomico-pathological study of 70 specimens (using a special technique) with particular reference to the problem of cervical spondylosis. Brain *80*, 571–596 (1957)

68. Pedersen, H.E., Blunck, C.F.J., Gardner, E.: The anatomy of lumbosacral posterior rami and meningeal branches of the spinal nerves (sinu vertebral nerves): with an experimental study of their function. J. Bone Jt Surg. (Amer.) *38*A, 377–391 (1956)

69. Picard, L., Roland, J., Blanchot, P., David, R., Montaut, J., Pourel, J.: Scarring of the theca and the nerve roots as seen at radiculography J. Neuroradiol. *4*, 29–48 (1977)

70. Renard, M., Masson, J.P., Larde, D.: Contribution à l'étude anatomo-radiologique du système veineux rachidien de la jonction lombo-sacrée. Bull. Assoc. Anat. (Fr.), *59*, 166, 725–735 (1975)

71. Roland, J., Larde, D., Masson, J.P., Picard, L.: Les veines lombaires épidurales. Radio-anatomie normale. J. Radiol. Electrol. *58* (1), 35–38 (1977)

72. Roland, J., Larde, D., Schwartz, J.F., Sigiel, M., Picard, L.: Intérêt de la phlébographie lombaire dans le diagnostic des discopathies lombaires. J. Radiol. Electrol. *57* (2), 175–182 (1976)

73. Rosenberg, N.J.: Dégénérative spondylolisthésis. J. Bone Jt Surg. (Amer.) *57* (4), 467–474 (1975)

74. Rousseau, R., Gournet, G.: Phlébographie rachidienne par voie transépineuse. Rev. Med. Nancy *81*, 377–384 (1956)

75. Rovira, M.O., Torrent, J., Ruscadella: Some aspects of the spinal cord circulation in cervical myelopathy. Neuroradiology *9*, 209–214 (1975)

76. Salamon, G., Louis, R., Guerinel, G.: Le fourreau dural lombosacré. Etude radio-anatomique. Acta Radiol. Diagn. *5*, 1107–1123 (1966)

77. Schobinger, R.A.: Intraosseous venography. New York: Grune and Stratton 1960

78. Schobinger, R., Lessmann, F.P.: A new approach allowing the roentgenologic demonstration of the cervical vertebral venous plexi. Exp. Med. Surg. *15*, 289–294 (1957)

79. Taylor, A.R.: Vascular factors in the myelopathy associated with cervical spondylosis. Neurology *14*, 62–68 (1964)

80. Theron, J.: Cervicovertebral phlebography: Pathological results. Radiology *118* (1), 73–81 (1976)

81. Theron, J.: Communication au Colloque d'Anatomie Radiologique et Biomécanique du Rachis, Montpellier (1976)

82. Theron, J., Djindjian, R.: Cervicovertebral phlebography using catheterization. A preliminary report. Radiology *108*, (2) 325–331 (1973)

83. Theron, J., Houtteville, J.P., Adam, H., Thurel, C., Rey, A., Loyau, G.: La phlébographie lombaire, aspect normal et intérêt dans le diagnostic des hernies discales. Rev. Rhum. Mal. Ostéoartic. *44*, 3, 165–171 (1977)

84. Theron, J., Houtteville, J.P., Ammerich, H., Alves De Souza, A., Adam, H., Thurel, C., Rey, A., Houdart, R.: Lumbar phlebography by catheterization of the lateral sacral and ascending lumbar veins with abdominal compression. Neuroradiology *11*, 175–182 (1976)

85. Theron, J., Tournade, A., Thurel, C., Rey, A., Chaye, M., Houtteville, J.P., Djindjian, R., Houdart, R.: La phlébographie lombaire. Communication Soc. de Neuroradiol. (1975)

86. Verbiest, H.: A radicular syndrome from developmental narrowing of the lumbar vertebral canal. J. Bone Jt Surg. (Brit.) *36*, 230–237 (1954)

87. Verbiest, H.: Fallacies of the present definition, nomenclature, and classification of the stenoses of the lumbar vertebral canal. Spine *1* (4), 217–225 (1976)

88. Verbiest, H., Paz Y Geuse, H.D.: Anterolateral surgery for cervical spondylosis in cases of myelopathy or nerve-root compression. J. Neurosurg. *25*, 611–622 (1966)

89. Vignaud, J., Moret, J., Faures, B., Chaouat, Y.: La phlébographie rachidienne lombaire. Son application en pathologie lombo-radiculaire. Rev. Rhum. Mal. Ostéoartic. *41*, 441–447 (1974)

90. Vogelsang, H.: Intraosseous Spinal Venography. Amsterdam: Excerpt. Med. 1970

91. Wackenheim, A., Babin, E.: Sténoses et Etroitesses du Canal Rachidien Lombaire. Journées nationales de radiologie. Cours de perfectionnement post-universitaire, Paris (16 Nov. 1977)

92. Wilkinson, M.: Cervical Spondylosis. Philadelphia: Saunders 1971

Subject Index

Vein
lumbar   33, 35, 38, 39, 112
medial epidural cervical   123, 126, 127
medial epidural lumbar   29, 30, 48, 49, 51
of the lateral foramen   28, 29, 31, 46, 47,
    43, 122
posterior condyloid   119
radicular   62, 115, 127
spinal   150

subclavian   123
vertebral   119, 122, 123
Vena cava
inferior   3, 4, 33, 35, 43
superior   3, 33, 123
Vertebral artery   4, 122, 143
Vertebral plexus   122

Xenon   5

Angiography of the Human Brain Cortex

Atlas of Vascular Patterns and Stereotactic Cortical Localization
By G. Szikla, G. Bouvier, T. Hori, V. Petrov
With the collaboration of E. A. Cabanis,
P. Farnarier, M. T. Iba-Zizen
Foreword by J. Talairach

1977. 22 figures, 199 plates. XII, 273 pages
Cloth DM 340,–; US $ 170.00
ISBN 3-540-08285-9
Distribution rights for Japan:
Maruzen Co. Ltd., Tokyo

H. V. Crock, H. Yoshizawa

The Blood Supply of the Vertebral Column and Spinal Cord in Man

1977. 120 figures, 44 color plates.
XIII, 130 pages
Cloth DM 98,–; US $ 49.00
ISBN 3-211-81402-7
Distribution rights for Japan:
Nankodo Co. Ltd., Tokyo

Y. Dirheimer

The Craniovertebral Region in Chronic Inflammatory Rheumatic Diseases

With a Foreword by A. Wackenheim

1977. 86 figures, 6 tables. XI, 173 pages
Cloth DM 98,–; US $ 49.00
ISBN 3-540-08160-7

R. Djindjian, J.-J. Merland

Super-Selective Arteriography of the External Carotid Artery

With the collaboration of J. Théron
Translated from the French by
I. F. Moseley. Preface by R. Houdart

1978. 1068 figures, 5 plates, some in colour. XVI, 550 pages
Cloth DM 430,–; US $ 215.00
ISBN 3-540-08118-6

H. M. Duvernoy

Human Brainstem Vessels

Foreword by R. Warwick
Illustrations by J. L. Vannson

1978. 108 figures, 2 folding plates.
IX, 188 pages
Cloth DM 290,–; US $ 145.00
ISBN 3-540-08336-7

Spinal Angiomas

Advances in Diagnosis and Therapy
Editors: H. W. Pia, R. Djindjian
1978. Approx. 230 figures, 40 tables.
Approx. 260 pages
Cloth DM 120,–; US $ 60.00
ISBN 3-540-08369-3
Distribution rights for Japan:
Maruzen Co. Ltd., Tokyo

A. Wackenheim, J. P. Braun

The Veins of the Posterior Fossa

Normal and Pathologic Findings
With a Foreword by J. Bull
1978. 171 figures. XI, 157 pages
Cloth DM 136,–; US $ 68.00
ISBN 3-540-08337-5

Preisänderungen vorbehalten

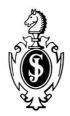

Springer-Verlag
Berlin Heidelberg New York

Springer Computerized Tomography

Clinical Computer Tomography

Head and Trunk
Editors: A. Baert, L. Jeanmart,
A. Wackenheim

1978. 414 figures, 2 tables. VIII, 261 pages
DM 78,–; US $ 39.00
ISBN 3-540-08458-4
Distribution rights for Japan:
Igaku Shoin Ltd., Tokyo

Computerized Axial Tomography

An Anatomic Atlas of Serial Sections
of the Human Body
Anatomy – Radiology – Scanner
By J. Gambarelli, G. Guérinel, L. Chevrot,
M. Mattèi
With the technical collaboration of
R. Galliano, S. Nazarian
Drawings by J. P. Jacomy. Photographies
by D. Amy, M. Soler

1977. 550 figures, some in color.
VI, 286 pages
Cloth DM 240,–; US $ 120.00
ISBN 3-540-07961-0

Cranial Computerized Tomography

Editors: W. Lanksch, E. Kazner
Editorial Board: T. Grumme, F. Marguth,
H. R. Müller, H. Steinhoff, S. Wende
1976. 620 figures. XIV, 478 pages
DM 78,–; US $ 39.00
ISBN 3-540-07938-6
Distribution rights for Japan:
Nankodo Co. Ltd., Tokyo

The Diagnostic Limitations of Computerised Axial Tomography

Editor: J. Bories
1978. 175 figures, 52 tables. IX, 220 pages
DM 54,–; US $ 27.00
ISBN 3-540-08593-9
Distribution rights for Japan:
Nankodo Co. Ltd., Tokyo

The First European Seminar on Computerised Axial Tomography in Clinical Practice

Editors: G. H. Du Boulay, I. F. Moseley
1977. 335 figures. XI, 430 pages
DM 78,–; US $ 39.00
ISBN 3-540-08116-X
Distribution rights for Japan:
Nankodo Co. Ltd., Tokyo

Preisänderungen vorbehalten

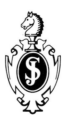

Springer-Verlag
Berlin Heidelberg New York